SEXUAL INTIMACY BETWEEN THERAPISTS AND PATIENTS

Sexual Medicine, Volume 5
HAROLD I. LIEF, M.D., SERIES EDITOR

VOLUMES IN THE SERIES

SEXUAL INTIMACY BETWEEN THERAPISTS AND PATIENTS

Kenneth S. Pope
Jacqueline C. Bouhoutsos

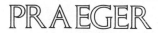

New York
Westport, Connecticut
London

RC
480.8
.P66
1986

Library of Congress Cataloging-in-Publication Data

Pope, Kenneth S.
  Sexual intimacy between therapists and patients.

  (Sexual medicine ; v.5)
  1. Psychotherapist and patient.   2. Psychotherapists
—Sexual behavior.   3. Psychotherapy patients—Sexual
behavior.   I. Bouhoutsos, Jacqueline C.   II. Title.
[DNLM: 1. Professional-Patient Relations.   2. Psycho-
therapy.   3. Sex Behavior.   4. Sex Offenses.
W1 SE99F v.5 / WM 62 P825s]
RC480.8.P66 1986   364.1 '68   86-15165
ISBN 0-275-92253-7 (alk. paper)
ISBN 0-275-92953-1 (pbk.: alk. paper)

Library of Congress Catalog Card Number: 86-15165

ISBN: 0-275-92253-7
        0-275-92953-1 (pbk.)

First published in 1986

Praeger Publishers, One Madison Avenue, New York, NY 10010
A division of Greenwood Press, Inc.

Printed in the United States of America

∞

The paper used in this book complies with the
Permanent Paper Standard issued by the National
Information Standards Organization (Z39.48-1984).

10   9   8   7   6   5   4   3   2

Foreword

The prohibition against physicians having sexual relations with patients is thousands of years old. The oath of Hippocrates is a clear injunction against sexual congress between the physician and the patient. It is equally unethical for mental health therapists of all types to have sexual contact with their patients. The injurious effects on patients of this form of sexual exploitation caused both the American Psychiatric Association and the American Psychological Association to revise their ethical codes specifically to prohibit sexual contact between therapists and patients.

As Pope and Bouhoutsos point out, sexual intimacy between therapists and patients received relatively little attention until the last decade or so. A number of surveys have demonstrated that this sort of therapeutic miscarriage occurs frequently enough to be a scandalous matter. A nationwide survey of psychiatrists, reported in May 1986, found that 6.4 percent of respondents acknowledged sexual contact with their patients. Three national surveys of psychologists reported a range of explicit sexual contact between male therapists and patients from 9.4 percent to 12.1 percent (2 to 3 percent of female therapists had been sexually intimate with their patients). Social workers reported a smaller prevalence rate. Surveys of marital, family, and sex therapists have not been reported, but there is no reason to anticipate that these professional groups would be very different from the three professions just cited.

This is a book for mental health professionals concerned about the moral, legal, and therapeutic aspects of the problem. It is the first comprehensive account of the motivations and personalities of the involved therapists and patients, the consequences for the actors in this painful and often sordid drama, and the difficulties encountered by therapists who attempt to repair the damage. The book includes three chapters dealing with the treatment of the patient sexually abused by a previous therapist. Pope and Bouhoutsos offer suggestions intended to help patients file complaints, as well as guidelines for lawyers and expert witnesses. A section dealing with prevention, providing checklists of warning signs for both patients and therapists, should prove to be most useful in warding off potential trouble.

The timing of this book is fortunate but hardly fortuitous. The mounting concern, the crescendo of criminal and civil lawsuits, the refusal of insurance carriers to protect therapists against liability created by allegations of sexual misconduct, the increasing number of studies reporting injurious consequences of therapist/patient sexual intimacy provided the background for the book and the motivations of the authors. Their scholarly approach is made eminently readable by the inclusion of many hypothetical and actual case histories. It is hardly necessary to enliven a topic of such intrinsic interest and attraction, and yet the authors have done just that. I welcome the opportunity to add this fifth volume to the series on Sexual Medicine.

Harold I. Lief, M.D.

Preface

The persistent denial regarding the topic of therapist-patient sexual intimacy has been a tragedy for the mental health professions and especially for the patients who were victimized by this unprofessional behavior. As is documented in the chapters that follow, the professions have begun to acknowledge and seriously address this phenomenon only in the last 15 or 20 years.

In this book we have attempted to draw together the currently available material on therapist-patient sexual intimacy from sources as diverse as clinical studies, first-person accounts, national surveys, legislation and case law, ethical standards, popular literature, as well as the evidence we ourselves have accumulated through our work as researchers and clinicians. We hope to make this information accessible to the widest possible audience; practicing clinicians; researchers; former, current, and prospective therapy patients; attorneys; educators; clinic administrators; legislators and policymakers; and the members of ethics committees and other professional review boards. We believe the information will be valuable not only in helping to alleviate the devastating trauma associated with sexual involvement between therapist and patient but also in the formulation of policies and standards, monitoring and regulatory mechanisms, resources to help "at risk" therapists to avoid sexually abusing their patients, and educational strategies that can serve to prevent what one former president of the American Psychological Association termed a "national disgrace."

We express our appreciation to Jay Ziskin, Karl Seuthe, and Catherine Seuthe, attorneys at law, for their review of and assistance with the sections pertaining to legal issues.

We also thank Michael Fisher, Medical Editor of Praeger Publishers, for the supportively enthusiastic approach with which he greeted our proposal for this book and the subsequent manuscript.

Finally, we wish formally to thank each other for the patience and collegiality that made the writing of this book a meaningful experience.

Contents

SEXUAL INTIMACY BETWEEN THERAPISTS AND PATIENTS

Varieties of Sexual Intimacy and How They Occur

AWARENESS OF COMMON SCENARIOS

Long a taboo topic, sexual intimacy between therapists and patients is still a painful topic for many of us. So devastating are the consequences for the patients and so deep is the betrayal of trust (let alone of laws, ethics, and professional standards) on the part of the therapist, that we tend to avert our eyes and act as if it never or rarely occurred. We engage in denial and discounting. We develop a habit of "selective inattention."

Yet the evidence, to be discussed in later chapters, indicates we are facing a major problem, one that a former president of the American Psychological Association termed the national disgrace of his profession. Therapist-patient sexual intimacy has become or is becoming the major source of complaints for many professional ethics committees. Numerous headlines document the proliferation of malpractice suits and actions by state licensing boards attempting—often unsuccessfully—to address this problem. In some national surveys, more than one out of ten male therapists report engaging in such intimacies with their patients.

The first step in successfully addressing this widespread problem is awareness. In what forms does therapist-patient sexual intimacy appear? How does it arise in the course of therapy? The answers to these questions are crucially important for the providers and consumers of mental health services.

For the therapist who has not yet engaged in sexual intimacies with patients, recognition that therapy is moving, however subtly and unintentionally, toward one of these scenarios can prompt timely and effective preventive measures. A careful review of the course of treatment, formal consultation with a colleague, perhaps reentering therapy are among the steps often helpful to a therapist who feels "at risk." Unfortunately, the taboo nature of sexual feelings about patients and the fear of damaging one's reputation by creating disapproval, doubts, or suspicions in the minds of colleagues makes it difficult for many therapists to consult their colleagues effectively about such issues. (Appendix A may be helpful to therapists who wish to explore these issues in a systematic manner.)

For the patient who feels that somethings is "not quite right" about the therapy, who is somehow anxious and concerned about sexual feelings or behavior in the therapeutic situation, awareness of these scenarios can help him or her make an effective exploration and informed decision about the propriety of the current treatment. (Appendix B may be a useful guide to such exploration.) Sexual thoughts, feelings, fantasies, as well as fear, shame, and guilt about sexual impulses, arousal, memories, or intentions are not uncommon themes in psychotherapy. They often create in patients reactions of acute discomfort and vulnerability. Deciding whether the therapy is a useful exploration or a subtle exploitation of these themes can be difficult under the best of circumstances. Knowledge of the common scenarios of therapist-patient sexual involvement can provide alerting signs, prompting patients to address directly issues of trust, *informed* consent to treatment, and the safety and integrety of the therapeutic process. Raising such concerns with the therapist and often with consultants (to get a "second opinion" from a new perspective) is a necessary step. What is hard for many patients is to avoid pushing such concerns back out of awareness, perhaps by reflexively labeling them "transference," "projection," "chronic suspicion," "resistance," "desire to avoid talking about sex," and so on. This superficial labeling—which shuts off rather than encourages thoughtful and honest exploration—is often aided and abetted by the therapist who can supply authoritative-sounding and intimidating technical jargon. Of course, the concerns may indeed reflect other issues active in the treatment. The point is to arrive at an understanding of the concerns and what is prompting them through careful, open, and informed consideration rather than through impulsive, reflexive denial, dismissal, or labeling.

An awareness of common scenarios for therapist-patient sexual intimacy can also be useful for the subsequent therapists of both patients and therapists who have been involved in such intimacies. For patients, the healing process often involves difficult and protracted attempts to understand how the involvement occurred and to deal with the characteristic feelings of guilt, ambivalence, and so on, vis-a-vis the exploitive therapist. For therapists, attempts at rehabilitation often involve both education regarding therapist-patient sexual intimacy (how it generally occurs, the devastating effects, the risk factors, and so on) and a more personal effort to set aside the numerous rationalizations and distortions in order to acknowledge, accept, and understand the event as it actually took place. Just as those who sexually abuse children, who rape, or who batter spouses often maintain a mythology about how the recipient of such violence and abuse "asked for it," "needed it," "was seductive," "deserved it," and may be better off for it, so also does the offending therapist often maintain a personal belief system that points the finger of blame and responsibility at the patient.

Awareness of these scenarios is important for professional organizations and educational institutions. Both providers and consumers of therapeutic services need comprehensive and continuing education about activities that lead to clearly unethical and clinically damaging sexual intimacies.

Finally, there may be some therapists, currently engaging in sexual activity with their patients, who may recognize themselves and their behavior in these scenarios. Whatever the reasons they have allowed this stituation to develop, the shock of recognition or the framework for understanding the implications of their behavior may enable them to take prompt action to discontinue the sexual involvement and to bring about the most constructive resolution. Finding the courage and integrity to initiate such action, in the absence of external pressure (such as lawsuits, complaints with licensing boards, and such), may prevent further damage to the patients and constitute a significant step in the rehabilitation of the therapist.

COMMON SCENARIOS OF THERAPIST-PATIENT SEXUAL INTIMACY

The scenarios presented in this section are based upon the clinical and research literature, public records (for example, transcripts of civil suits and administrative hearings), and our own professional study of this area. Most instances of therapist-patient sexual intimacy tend to fall into ten general scenarios—although there are, of course, many exceptions—each with its own dynamics and likely course of development (see Table 1). Our intention is to provide the salient aspects of each scenario while respecting the privacy of those—particularly patients—involved. Therefore the examples of the ten common scenarios are fictional generalizations, and none refers to a specific individual case.

Role Trading

Example

Amy is a 21-year-old college student who found Bob, her new therapist, by looking in the Yellow Pages under "Social Work." She is quite anxious as she begins to tell him of the problems she is having with her boyfriend. She is much too ashamed to open up about her parents, about the fights, the heavy drinking, and the occasional violence.

TABLE 1. Ten Common Scenarios

Scenario	Criterion
1. Role Trading	Therapist becomes the "patient" and the wants and needs of the therapist become the focus.
2. Sex Therapy	Therapist fraudulently presents therapist-patient sexual intimacy as a valid treatment for sexual or other kinds of difficulties.
3. As If . . .	Therapist treats positive transference as if it were not the result of the therapeutic situation.
4. Svengali	Therapist creates and exploits an exaggerated dependence on the part of the patient.
5. Drugs	Therapist uses cocaine, alcohol, or other drugs as part of the seduction.
6. Rape	Therapist uses physical force, threats, and/or intimidation.
7. True Love	Therapist uses rationalizations that attempt to discount the clinical/professional nature of the relationship with its attendant responsibilities.
8. It Just Got Out of Hand	Therapist fails to treat the emotional closeness that develops in therapy with sufficient attention, care, and respect.
9. Time Out	Therapist fails to acknowledge and take account of the fact that the therapeutic relationship does not cease to exist between scheduled sessions or outside the therapist's office.
10. Hold Me	Therapist exploits patient's desire for nonerotic physical contact and possible confusion between erotic and nonerotic contact.

Bob is sympathetic. He wishes to put her at ease, to assure her that such problems are not out of the ordinary. To help her overcome here feelings of isolation, he begins sharing (modeling self-disclosure) something of his own life, of the problems he is having with his wife, the "family secrets" with which he's had to live.

Amy is reassured and fascinated. She wants to hear more about his life, about how he handled problems similar to the ones she is facing. Bob obliges. He begins going into more and more detail about the lack of communication in his marriage, his wife's lack of interest in him, the sexual problems resulting from his wife's vaginismus.

Amy and Bob begin to discover that they have a great deal in common. Amy looks forward to each session and asks if they can increase the frequency of their visits. She finds her self-esteem improving because Bob treats her like an adult (something neither her parents nor her boyfriend ever did). She feels more worthwhile because she is able to understand Bob's problems and to help him with them, sometimes only by listening to him and "being there." Her own problems, the one's that led her to seek therapy, seem less important; she no longer feels very connected to her family or her boyfriend. She is finding a new relationship, of a kind that feels very natural to her, in which she is grounded. For the first time in her life, she feels truly special.

Bob agrees to the increased sessions and notes Amy's improvement in his otherwise sparse treatment records. He finds himself looking forward to their sessions. He decides that his theoretical orientation is not really analytic, but rather existential-humanistic. His "authenticity" with Amy is obviously therapeutic. Their ability to be "real" with each other is enabling her to be more "whole," to experience herself as valuable and alive.

Soon they are meeting five days a week and Bob discovers that, for the first time in his life, he feels truly understood. He begins opening himself up to feelings he never knew he had. When he is most vulnerable, Amy is always there with just the right word of understanding and reassurance. During one session he becomes so profoundly moved when talking about the pain he experienced as a young child, of never being held in a safe embrace, Amy comes over and hugs him. He puts his arms around her and they feel a special closeness.

After the session in which they hugged each other, the customary arrangement—Bob sitting in his chair, Amy on the couch—began to seem stilted, inauthentic, out of touch with the reality of their closeness. They moved to the couch, where Bob would often lie with his head in her lap, she comforting him while he told her more and more about himself, things he had never told anyone.

One day Bob told her he was going to take the greatest risk of his life and tell her his deepest secret. With much difficulty, he told her that his deepest wish was to make love with a real woman, and that the only real woman he knew was Amy. Amy cared for Bob in a way she had cared for no one else, in a way that she had always wished someone would care for her. She told him that there was nothing she wouldn't do for him.

Discussion

In the same way that in some disturbed family patterns (often involving incest and similar role and boundary disturbances) the children become "parents" to their own parents, trying to please and take care of them, some disturbed therapy patterns involve a reversal of roles. The patient's role is to care for, please, and gratify the wants and needs of the therapist. The slippery slope toward sexual intimacy often begins with gradual, almost imperceptible trends. The therapist becomes the talker, the patient the listener. The life and needs of the therapist become the focus. The legitimate needs of the patient become secondary or denied altogether. The patient begins feeling special and important as a result of his or her obvious importance to the therapist. The patient will feel responsible for the depression, guilt, frustration, tiredness, and other problems communicated by the therapist. Sexually gratifying the therapist is but one of the many ways in which the patient fulfills this function.

This pattern stresses the crucial necessity of all therapists ensuring that they have adequate resources for gratifying their own wants and needs *outside* of their relationships with their patients. If therapists are experiencing difficulties in their personal lives, consultation, supervision, and/or (re)entering therapy are useful, if not absolutely necessary, steps to prevent damage to their work with patients.

Sex Therapy

Example

Cathy is a patient of Dr. Donald, a charismatic psychiatrist. She complains of not experiencing orgasm during intercourse. Dr. Donald begins by taking a careful history, including a sexual history, and notes that among Cathy's difficulties is a feeling of shame about her body. She fears that it is not attractive and thus is anxious when she removes her clothes to make love.

Dr. Donald explains that the first phase of treatment involves two techniques that the medical literature terms "reality testing" and "systematic desensitization." He refers to prestigious scientific journals in which these techniques are discussed and assures her that they are not only legitimate approaches but also are quite necessary if she is ever to overcome her problem. Cathy feels uneasy when the doctor explains what she must do, but, after all, he is a licensed physician and she desperately wants to be cured.

He begins by asking her to remove her blouse and to report to him when she first begins to experience the anxiety. For several sessions, Cathy is unable even to unbutton her blouse, but Dr. Donald works persistently and carefully with this resistance, pointing out that it is a normal aspect of her difficulty and of the process of therapy. On the fourth session, she removes her blouse. Dr. Donald comments that she has made a significant step toward improvement.

The next session he asks her to remove both her blouse and her bra. The "resistance" associated with this phase of "treatment" lasts two more sessions.

During the session when she has finally removed all the garments from her upper body, Dr. Donald looks at her with a professional manner and states that the systematic desensitization is progressing well, that she now seems able to experience her anxiety and to deal with it more effectively. He then explains that he will begin commenting on his impressions of her body so that she will have professional judgment to use in her "reality testing." In this way she can come to have a more realistic view of her body and its attractiveness.

The course of "therapy" proceeds to involve her removing all of her clothes, to deal with the resistance and anxiety associated with that behavior, and to "be open" to Dr. Donald's comments about her body.

Having successfully completed this phase of her "therapy," Cathy now listens to the doctor explain that the first step in evaluating her difficulty experiencing orgasms will involve seeing under what conditions she currently has no difficulty. During the history, she had explained that her difficulty was only during intercourse, not during masturbation.

Dr. Donald explains that they must now explore her orgasmic capability. She must lie on the floor and masturbate to climax. Resistance to this phase lasts two months. However, the doctor's calm and reassuring manner, combined with his increasingly authoritative statements that she absolutely must follow the treatment plan in order to "get well" causes Cathy to set aside her doubts again and to "follow the doctor's orders."

Twice while attempting to comply, she bursts into tears, dresses hurriedly, and rushes out of his office. But soon she is able to complete the exercise, finding that Dr. Donald talks to her the whole time to help her with her "reality testing." During one session Dr. Donald lies down on the floor close to her, "in order to give her reassurance and to observe what is really causing your problem." Soon he is touching her. She is confused and frightened, but also sexually excited. They engage in intercourse. That afternoon she jumps off the top of an office building near her home.

Discussion

The factors that therapists have at their disposal to manipulate patients into overriding their doubts about and resistance to sexual involvement are numerous and varied. Patients are often confused and anxious about their sexuality and thus vulnerable to influence. There is the common desire, sometimes almost a compulsion, to please the therapist. There is the confusion related to the transference phenomenon. There is the control and license we grant to doctors: we allow some kinds of doctors to put us to sleep and to cut into us, others to inject us with potentially lethal chemicals, still others to examine us when we are naked and to probe the private parts of our bodies. There is the authority of doctors. Despite the healthy skepticism of the consumer movement and our deeply ingrained love-hate relationship to the medical-professional establishment, there are few of us who do not harbor a hopeful belief that "the doctor knows best." There is the desperation of intensely distressing and disabling conditions that make the patient ready to "try anything" in order to feel better. Moreover, as important as any of the others, there is the fact that a deep trust is a crucially important aspect of any therapeutic relationship. This trust makes the patient extremely vulnerable to the therapist.

As If . . .

Example

Ellen was disconcerted when she discovered, in only her third session with Frank, a clinical psychologist, that she was attracted to him. She viewed this as the worst possible thing that could happen. She had wanted to discuss, among other concerns, some issues involving her relationships with men, and now here she was developing a crush on her therapist. How could she work on these other problems if she fell in love with Frank? And how could she possibly face the embarassment of telling him her secret? He'd probably get angry with her and tell her that he couldn't work with her. Or he'd just laugh at her, and she'd still be stuck with her feelings.

She hoped that by ignoring the problem it would go away. After several weeks it got worse. She found herself dreaming about him, and once even became aware of a sexual fantasy about him. During the sessions she would try to talk about the problems that had prompted her to enter therapy, but she found herself imagining the two of them doing all sorts of things together.

She became more resolute in her efforts to block these thoughts out of her mind. Nevertheless, she found herself becoming sexually excited at the mere thought of going to therapy and when she was sitting with him in the quiet intimacy of his office, it was all she could do to control herself. During one session, while he was talking, she lapsed into a vivid sexual fantasy and found herself so intensely excited that she felt close to orgasm. Frank noticed that she was quite flushed and asked if anything was wrong. She shook her head and said, "Nothing."

The situation had become intolerable for her. During her therapist's vacation she decided that she must do something. She felt she was being driven crazy by her thoughts. She gathered her courage and resolved that, no matter what embarrassment she felt and no matter how angry or ridiculing Frank might respond, she would talk about what was going on with her. If she could at least talk about it, bring it out into the open, then she and Frank could decide what to do about it. After all, perhaps it was normal for some patients to fall in love with their therapists, though she wasn't really sure if she truly believed that. Even if it wasn't normal, they could make it one of the issues she would deal with in therapy. Maybe it was somehow related to the other problems she'd been trying to deal with. Of course it was possible, given the intensity of her feelings, that she just wouldn't be able to work with Frank. This worried her. But she would have to face it, and maybe he would help her to find a new therapist with whom she'd be able to work more effectively.

Once she made the decision to bring the matter out into the open she was nervous, but somehow she felt that a huge weight had been lifted from her. During the days while she waited for Frank to return from vacation, she found that she wasn't dreaming about him so much, that she became sexually excited when thinking about him much less often and much less intensely. In fact, she began to have more specific ideas about how her infatuation with him was similar to feelings she had had about her ex-husband and the men with whom she'd been involved after the divorce. These relationships had always ended up causing her so much pain, and now she felt more hopeful that she might be able to figure out what she found attractive about such men and how she got involved with them.

As she took the elevator up to Frank's office for her first session after his vacation, she was aware that for the first time in many weeks she was not sexually excited when she approached the session. She was still somewhat nervous but felt confident and sure of herself, eager to see how much work they could do.

When Ellen began talking about how attracted she'd been to him, Frank found himself paying intense attention. He had found her among the most beautiful and intelligent, let alone intriguing, women he had ever met. Now it turned out she was in love with him. The idea excited him beyond belief. He watched her shift positions in her chair and found his body stirring. He began breathing deeply and knew that his face was flushed.

Ellen was so much more vibrant than his current lover, with whom he'd become somewhat bored. Now she was not only telling him that she was in love with him but she was describing some sexual fantasies she'd had about him. This could be, he thought, the perfect relationship. She was saying something about how she'd always fantasized that he'd come over and kiss her. Impulsively he interrupted her. "Stand up." "What?" she asked. He repeated, louder, "Stand up!"

Having no idea what was happening, she stood up, wondering if he was going to order her out of his office. Though she'd almost forgotten it, one of her original fears had been that if she confessed these feelings he would abandon her.

Immediately when she stood up, he went over and put his arms around her and tried to kiss her. She struggled to get away but was confused. Her mind became blurry and she felt as if she were going to faint. There was nothing she wanted more at that moment than to be out of that office, out of that situation, dead if that is what it would take.

"You want this," he said, holding her tight, pawing at her, shoving her clothes aside. She began to cry and tried with all her strength to push him away. He seemed passionate and angry at her. Her mind ceased to function effectively. Years later, even with intensive psychotherapy to aid her recovery, she found it impossible to think of this experience without terror, nausea, and shame. Her sexual relationship with this therapist will be the single most destructive event in her life.

Discussion

For most of us, there is something deeply pleasing when others tell us that they find us sexually appealing, are romantically attracted to us, are falling in love with us. It can make us flattered and proud. It can make us feel accepted and affirmed. It can make us feel validated, privileged, special. The list of positive reactions is varied and almost limitless. At times it may make for some awkward moments, it may elicit conflicts, it may complicate our lives, but generally we like being told.

One of the best things about being told that someone is attracted to us is that we take it personally. It says something—at least we like to think it does—about us as unique individuals. That's perhaps the heart of the problem in the therapeutic relationship.

In the therapeutic relationship the patient, through transference and a host of related phenomena, can experience powerful feelings of sexual attraction for the therapist that are not essentially related to the therapist as an individual. There is nothing out of the ordinary or antitherapeutic about the occurrence and verbal expression of such feelings. Indeed, their occurrence and the efforts to accept and understand them may constitute the essential work of many therapies.

It is the therapist's responsibility to recognize such feelings as essentially different from those that might occur outside the therapeutic relationship, and to handle them responsibly. This principle has been clearly and explicitly established at least as early as Freud's statement in 1915 that the patient's transference must be placed in a different context than "falling in love" as it develops in nontherapeutic relationships. The analyst "must recognize that the patient's falling in love is induced by the analytic situation and is not to be ascribed to the charms of his person, that he has no reason whatsoever therefore to be proud of such of 'conquest', as it would be called outside analysis" (Freud 1963, p. 169).

Therapists commit a serious error with damaging consequences when they respond to clients' sexual attraction as if it occurred in a different context. These "As If . . ." scenarios are among the most confusing for both therapist and patient, and are among the most damaging.

Svengali

Example

Gilda is a charismatic counselor who demands total compliance from her patients. Heather, who has almost always had trouble "making my own decisions and running my own life," feels that Gilda is the perfect therapist for her. Always baffled by the complexities and demands of life, Heather finds that Gilda possesses knowledge and certainty for which she has always been searching.

Gilda helps her patients achieve their true potential by unfolding for them the mysteries of life and by instructing them in the correct way to live. She makes decisions for them in all aspects of their lives and will tolerate no resistance. She has a number of techniques—such as ridicule, intimidation, and threats of abandonment—for enlisting the trust and loyalty of her followers, but mainly she rules through the force of her personality. She lets them know what a unique and valuable service she is providing to her patients, and in her more reflective moments she has been known to compare herself to Socrates, Moses, Jesus, Buddha, and Albert Schweitzer.

She tells Heather that she is her favorite and that she has it in her to achieve almost unlimited goals if only she will open herself up to new experiences, to the wisdom that is available to her. She touches Heather frequently, putting her arm around her, stroking her hair, hugging her.

Heather gives herself over more and more to her therapist. She abides by her therapist's teachings in all areas of her life. It is as if she now derives her identity and will from Gilda.

Gilda informs Heather that she is now ready to receive the most sacred wisdom, the true communion of knowledge and spirit. Heather has difficulty understanding exactly what Gilda is talking about, but this is not new. Gilda has made it clear to her patients that it is often not possible or important for them to understand why they are doing something, only that they do it when she says it is in their interests. Understanding will come later, if at all, after they have opened themselves to the new experience.

Gilda soon makes Heather her lover.

Discussion

Svengalis, who often become intimate with numerous patients, are most often smoothly charming or powerfully authoritarian therapists. Charisma and mystique are crucial.

They find it most easy to exploit patients with marked dependency needs and a tendency to comply. Those who fear and respect authority are especially vulnerable. However, they have a wide range of techniques for imposing their will upon patients, and in many cases these techniques are similar to those used in brainwashing and hypnotism. They become gods to their patients, whose ability to think for themselves becomes acutely attenuated. Cults and cult-like customs and behavior are not uncommon. The sexual intimacy between therapist and patient may take on the trappings of a religious ritual, and may eventually involve three or more people.

Drugs

Example

Ivan, a therapist specializing in body work, is explaining to Jack, his new patient, what he is learning just by touching his body. The tightness in the shoulders, for example, shows the tension and strain he has been living under. "You're almost certainly not making as much money as you'd like and there are times that your work is not fulfilling to you. Sometimes you wonder if you've gone into the wrong line of work, but you are somewhat afraid of trying out new possibilities that might not work out." The curvature of the spine indicates deep-rooted feelings of inferiority, probably springing from childhood experiences they would need to explore in future sessions. "There are times you've been nervous about meeting new people or about being in a group of people. You feel inadequate in some ways, but sometimes it's difficult to talk about your inadequacies and sometimes it's hard even to admit them to yourself. There are some things about your body and about your self that you'd like to change." The slightly tilted line of the pelvis expresses sexual hang-ups that need prompt attention. "You've had some sexual experiences that didn't work out, some, in fact, were quite painful for you psychologically. You've had some fantasies about sexual activities that you haven't actually tried and some you believe you wouldn't want to try out. Sometimes you've been with someone—a sexual partner—and haven't done some of the sexual acts you would've liked. Sometimes you've felt rejected by a lover or someone to whom you've been sexually attracted. There are some ways in which you think your sex life could be different, might be improved.''

Ivan has already explained that his technique of body-mind integration is derived from his study of the work of Freud, Ferenczi, Reich, Lowen, Rolf, Feldenkrais, Janov, and Alexander. Colonics, rebirthing, and past-life regression are also among his resources. Yet Jack is still dumbfounded that a virtual stranger, no matter how well-informed and talented, could tell so much about him simply by having him disrobe and touching him. Of course, he is unaware that Ivan says virtually the same thing to all new patients, with very little variation.

During the second session, Ivan presents his patient with a detailed treatment plan that will begin with methods to relax Jack's "character armor" so that they may both discover the hidden pain and "engrams" throughout his body and begin to restructure a more positive development of body and mind. Deep massage will be a part of the treatment as will colonics, which rid the body of toxins. Ivan explains that the process of "disarmoring" can be considerably accelerated through the prudent use of safe, naturally occurring substances that have often been used by ancient cultures to enhance understanding and the sense of well-being. In our culture, Ivan explains, this substance is often referred to as cocaine, without a true appreciation of its therapeutic qualities. Ivan has assured Jack that he is a licensed physician and has been authorized to prescribe cocaine in his healing work. Nonetheless, he cautions Jack not to speak to others of this approach since Ivan fears he would be besieged by those seeking treatment for whom such approaches would not be beneficial.

The effects of the cocaine, in combination with the colonic and the constant touching, make Jack extremely vulnerable to sexual exploitation by his therapist.

Discussion

Drugs can be used by therapists in a variety of ways to implement a seduction. Some drugs tend to create a sense of heightened sexual sensitivity or arousal in some people. Some psychotropic medications impair the perceptual or motor processes, alertness, or ability to respond effectively. Some induce an almost comatose condition during which the patient is completely helpless. In still other instances a therapist may supply a drug that creates a strong psychological or chemical dependence. Once the patient becomes "hooked," the therapist can make sexual intimacies a condition for further "prescriptions."

Rape

Example

Karen is a 14-year-old victim of incest. Dr. Louis, a hypnotherapist, is treating her for the incest trauma. He makes her lie on his couch and attempts to put her in a deep trance. She is so nervous that she is unable to concentrate on what he is saying. She does not trust him, does not want to be seeing him, and lies on the couch, her face covered by her hands, crying.

He says it looks as if she needs reassurance, and he lies down next to her. He tells her she has nothing to be afraid of, that he will protect her and comfort her. He presses himself against her and, before she can scream, puts his hand over her mouth. He holds her so that she can neither cry or nor move. He rapes her.

When he is finished he tells her it never happened, that she is crazy and imagined the whole thing. He tells her that if she tries to tell anyone that no one will believe her. Everyone will believe that she is psychotic and needs to be put away in a hospital. If she tries to tell anyone, they will know that she was just making up stories about the incest, so they will either return her to her father or put her in jail. No matter where they put her, he will still be in charge of her treatment and they will always believe a famous hypnotherapist rather than a hysterical little girl who is always making up fantastic stories that show what a dirty mind she has. He may even tell them that she tried to seduce him and told him that she had made up the stories about the incest because she had been unable to seduce her father. He told her that if she tried to tell anyone what she had imagined had happened, that he would prescribe drugs that would make her a vegetable and might operate on her brain. If he felt like it, he might arrange for her to die. As she got dressed to leave, he slapped her to stop her from crying. He told her not to be late for their next appointment.

Discussion

As is obvious from the clinical theory and research cited in this book, the forceful transference phenomenon, the power differential between therapist and patient, the deep trust necessary to an effective therapeutic relationship, and similar factors significantly diminish a patient's ability to resist sexual advances. On this basis, Masters and Johnson (1976) have argued that therapists who use their power to engage in sexual intimacies with patients should be charged with rape. In this sense, all sexual intimacy within the context of a therapeutic relationship constitutes a form of rape. Nevertheless, in some instances, therapists may rely predominantly upon physical force, often involving considerable violence, to achieve sexual gratification with their patients. Thus the destructive consequences of rape accomplished through brute physical force and actual violence are compounded with the violation of the therapeutic relationship.

True Love

Example

In the second year of her analysis, Martha found herself strongly attracted to Dr. Nolls. As if by a stroke of destiny, Dr. Nolls looked within himself and discovered similar feelings for her. This was no sudden and superficial attraction, he told himself with conviction. For over a year he had given her his undivided attention for an hour a day, five days a week. He felt that he knew her better than he knew most of his friends. But it was more than that. In his work with her, he experienced a closeness, an intense intimacy that he had never felt before. He felt that they were soul-mates, brought together by fate. It was the most special relationship of his life.

For the next two months he pondered the dilemma, and he found himself talking more than he usually did during the analytic hour. Martha was responsive, and the discussion became more two-sided than before.

He didn't really know what to do. On the one hand, he had always believed that therapist-patient sex was an unacceptable practice. Yet this, somehow, was different, was special. He was no dirty old man, waiting to jump on a vulnerable patient; and she was no helpless victim, unable to choose what she wanted in life. She had her problems, but so did everyone. She was sophisticated, well-integrated, and had achieved a developmental level that was probably above average, even for those who were nonpatients. Her analysis was not really treatment in the traditional sense, he decided, but rather a means she used to explore new vistas, much as one might attend a seminar or keep an introspective diary. So she wasn't really a patient per se. She was more a fellow human being, someone with whom he enjoyed working.

There was more to it than that. Their feelings for each other were not the run-of-the-mill attraction. This was a once-in-a-lifetime pairing of two perfectly matched souls. The restrictions—clinical, ethical, legal—forbidding therapist-patient romances didn't really apply here. There's simply no rule that fits every person in every situation all the time. Martha and he were a special exception. What, after all, is more important, more special, more sacred than this rare kind of love? Could he ever justify casting aside this gift of life on the basis of rules written somewhere that didn't really apply to this sort of situation anyway?

His mind decided, he began one session by asking her not to recline on the couch but rather to sit facing him so that they could talk. He began by informing her that his feelings for her were as strong as hers for him. He was resolved not to handle the matter impulsively though he did mention the possibility of marriage somewhere down the line. He explained to her the necessity of dealing with their affair discreetly given the lack of understanding among the professional community and the public about their "special" situation. He mentioned the importance of maintaining, should their liaison ever become known to others, that the treatment was terminated before the affair was initiated. To facilitate this arrangement, he had written chart notes leading up to and through the successful termination and back-dated them by several months. Thus it would be clear to anyone that the therapy had been over for quite a while before they started seeing each other socially. He suggested a plan by which they would "accidentally" run into each other at a party some months hence, and would pretend that it was the first time they had seen each other since termination.

When he finished talking, they were only 20 minutes into the session. Since they still had more than a half hour left, they decided to move to the couch to get to know each other better and to share their joy.

Discussion

The inventive mind of the therapist need never run short of rationalizations for engaging in unprincipled behavior. "True love" is among the most powerful, seductive, and chronic of these justifications. Once the therapist is convinced of the presence of this special condition, all possible objections fall helpless before its awesome and mysterious sway. True love is its own justification and a seeming justification for all things. It makes "all fair." Like the Loreli, it lures the therapy off course toward untold destruction. It is only later when the spell fades, that the true horror of the consequences begin to make themselves known.

It Just Got Out of Hand

Example

Oliver was intelligent, handsome, physically strong yet emotionally sensitive. He was extremely shy and seemed to have a melancholy air about him, as if he were always preoccupied with something that had gone wrong sometime in the past. Nonetheless, he was a very successful businessman and managed to handle social situations well by masking his innate shyness with a marvellous sense of humor. Paula, his therapist, never quite felt she could arrive at an adequate diagnosis or a solid treatment plan, but she did her best to listen carefully to him and make helpful comments. Once or twice she considered referring him to another therapist, since something seemed to be interfering with her normally acute clinical intuition and ability to make timely interventions. But she found that she liked this patient a great deal and hoped that her unconditional positive regard for him would be therapeutic in itself and would eventually lead to a better formulation. Oliver, after all, seemed to be eager to work with her.

Oliver's business responsibilities seemed to be weighing more heavily on him. He was at the office almost all the time, having little opportunity to go home by a reasonable hour. Once he called her, said he was in crisis, and asked if she could come to his office to help "put him back together" before a crucial negotiation that would take place there in an hour and a half. He didn't feel he was in any shape to drive and, in any event, there was no way he could make it to her office and back in time for the negotiation and still have enough time to talk. Paula deliberated briefly before agreeing to meet him at his office. She felt it showed a healthy development of their working relationship that he could reach out to her in this crisis.

During the following month she met him twice more at his office. The latter time they decided to continue the session over dinner since neither of them had eaten. Paula saw no harm in that.

A landmark in Oliver's therapy was his decision to take a risk and open a branch office. He professed heartfelt and effusive thanks to Paula, telling her that without her support it would not have been possible. He said it would be very important and meaningful if she would attend the formal reception to celebrate the opening of the new office. She felt it was important to validate his growth and achievement so she agreed. As soon as she arrived, Oliver greeted her and escorted her around for the entire two hours. Afterward they went out to dinner to discuss what this had meant to him. He ordered a bottle of champagne and then another. He talked about how much this therapy had meant to him, how much she meant to him. He took her hand and told her that she was the most special person in his life. As she later described to her own therapist how she had come to spend the night with her patient, all she could really come up with was the phrase, "It just got out of hand."

Discussion

Therapists and their patients not only work in close and private physical proximity but also share an intense emotional intimacy. This intimacy, often the lifeblood of the therapy, must be regarded with deep respect and handled with care. It is always the therapist's responsibility to see that roles are not confused, that the emotional closeness does not lead to sexual contact. Patients, for a variety of reasons, may seem to invite a social, romantic, or sexual relationship that is at odds with the work and goals of therapy. It is always important for therapists to be respectful, understanding, and accepting of the impulses that give rise to these "invitations" but to make sure that therapy is a safe place for authentic therapeutic work. Thus therapists must see that they do not participate with their patients in "acting out" these impulses. In this way patients are always free to express—verbally—impulses, wishes, fantasies, desires, and invitations of all sorts with no restrictions or censorship. The therapist, however, maintains a safe and secure environment free from the inappropriate mutual participation in destructive activities.

It is important to note that within many legitimate theoretical orientations, therapists may engage in activities that take them out of the office and into the day-to-day lives of their patients. For instance when discussing work with suicidal patients, Bruce Danto (Colt 1983, pp. 56-57), a former director of the Detroit Suicide Prevention Center and former president of the American Association of Suicidology, states:

> With these problems, you can't simply sit back in your chair, stroke your beard and say "All the work is done right here in my office with my magical ears and tongue." There has to be a time when you shift gears and become an activist. Support may involve helping a patient get a job, attending a graduation or play, visiting the hospital, even making house calls.

M. H. Stone (1982, pp. 270–271) provides a vivid example of a therapist who "meets" a patient outside the office:

> A schizophrenic woman of twenty-two had been hospitalized because of a psychotic episode following the breakup of a romantic relationship. She continuously vilified her therapist for "not caring" about her, as though there were no distinction between the therapist and the departed lover. One day, in a fit of pique, the patient escaped from the hospital. The therapist, upon hearing the news, got into her car and canvassed all the bars and social clubs in Greenwich Village which her patient was known to frequent. At about midnight, she found her patient and drove her back to the hospital. From that day forward, the patient grew calmer, less impulsive, and made rapid progress in treatment. Later, after making a substantial recovery, she told her therapist that all the interpretations during the first few weeks in the hospital meant very little to her. But after the "midnight rescue mission" it was clear, even to her, how concerned and sincere her therapist had been from the beginning.

The point is not that therapists should never, under any circumstances, meet their patients outside the office or become involved in their lives but rather that such interventions must always and only be undertaken: within the context of a sound theoretical orientation, based on a carefully considered treatment plan, and with special attention paid to ensuring that they do not encourage or lead to sexual intimacy.

Time Out

Example

Dr. Quincy's therapy group meets at his office every Wednesday night from 7:00 to 8:45. Two day after the twenty-second meeting of the group, one of the patients, Reve, calls and asks if she can meet with him privately to discuss a personal matter. Because of his busy schedule, he asks her to join him for his brief lunch break between his morning and afternoon patients.

She asks him to advise her on a business matter, whose details she did not wish to share in the group, especially since the matter did not concern the intense themes with which the group was currently dealing. They dispose of the matter quickly and spend the rest of the lunch hour in enjoyable conversation.

Two weeks later she calls again and soon they begin meeting regularly for lunch. Both of them notice the mutual attraction and within two months, Reve begins visiting Dr. Quincy at his home and engaging in heavy petting and fellatio. After three months of sexual involvement, Reve abruptly drops out of the therapy group and discontinues all involvement with her therapist. She moves to another city, and manages to hold herself together for two years, virtually wiping out all active memory of her intimacy with Dr. Quincy. Over a course of the next year, she gradually begins to decompensate and loses her job. She is hospitalized after a psychotic break. Discharged from the hospital, she begins a long course of therapy and, after three years of work, becomes able to acknowledge the devastating impact her sexual involvement with her therapist had caused. For another two years she works on this issue in therapy and at that time decides she wishes to file a formal complaint against Dr. Quincy.

In responding to the complaint, Dr. Quincy attempts to deny that his involvement with Reve was in any way inappropriate, unethical, or illegal. First of all, he maintains, there was no intercourse, and therefore whatever occurred could not be termed "sexual intimacy." Second, whatever occurred never happened during the therapy sessions. Third, whatever occurred never took place at his office. Fourth, during whatever occurred, they never discussed her treatment. Thus it had nothing to do with her treatment, and had no impact on it whatsoever. Whatever occurred and Reve's treatment were entirely separate and unrelated. The licensing board revoked Dr. Quincy's license.

Discussion

Therapists can be amazingly resourceful in their attempts to create technical exceptions to the clear and thorough prohibitions against engaging in sexual intimacies with patients. They may try to build a wall between the therapy and the sexual intimacy based on spatial, temporal, or content distinctions. No longer able to argue convincingly that sexual intimacies are "therapeutic," they may now attempt to argue that sexual intimacies are not sexual intimacies. Like immature adolescents, they attempt to soothe their consciences (or, failing a conscience, public opinion) by saying that the most intimate, hot, and heavy activity is permissible as long as you don't "go all the way."

Hold Me

Example

Steve thought of himself as a remarkably insightful and sensitive therapist and Theresa, his patient, liked him because he was so warm and gentle. Not at all like her mother, who was so cold and distant. Ever since her mother had died a year ago, Theresa had felt utterly alone in the world. (Her father had left home when she was three.)

During the last two years of her life, Theresa had engaged in a series of brief and disastrous love affairs, and had entered therapy with the hope of making a better life for herself. She had never dreamed that she'd find such an understanding and accepting man as Steve.

As therapy progressed, she began to experience an intense longing to sit on his lap, to feel his strong arms wrapped around her, comforting her and protecting her from the world. It was hard for her to admit to him this overwhelming desire. She was surprised when he said that he could see nothing that would prevent her from doing just that. Though her deepest wish had just been made possible, she felt a strange anxiety.

When she hesitated, Steve, as usual, addressed her fears in a calm and reassuring voice. He told her that what they would be doing had a sound rationale. Therapy, he said, was often conceptualized by the best therapists as a "corrective emotional experience." Together they could recreate her childhood, but this time in a way that fostered healthy growth and development. He would be modeling for her a loving and accepting parent, so unlike the actual mother and father she'd had. He explained to her that one brilliant therapist had actually described the therapeutic situation as a "holding environment" and that his holding her would probably be the most therapeutic intervention. He told her about the concept of "overt transference," and how, in actually making her transference "real and authentic" in their behavior, it would be more clear and obvious as they attempted to deal with it. He even mentioned research showing how crucially important human touch is to normal human development.

When she finally sat in his lap, she found herself feeling as if she were a little baby. His stroking her hair and her back felt warm and good. Then he was stroking her legs. She grew dizzy and confused. She felt strange sensations and didn't know what to do about them. She felt a terror so profound that she was unable to move, unable to speak. It was as if she were in the nightmare where the monster is chasing her and she runs and runs but doesn't go anywhere. Her body became numb but she continued to hear his voice, soothing and hypnotic. He was saying something about wanting to be closer, of wanting to hold her without anything blocking their contact.

She left the office not really knowing what had happened. She became anxious and depressed, almost completely incapacitated between their sessions, overwhelmed and confused while she was with him. He kept telling her to trust him, that they had so many years of bad parenting to undo. She hated it when he undressed her and made her do things with him, but she felt it was the only way to have him hold her. When she was not being held by him, she felt as if she were disintegrating, as if she were empty, as if she didn't exist.

Discussion

In a number of cases, therapists exploit their patients' deep and overwhelming desire to be held and comforted. Sometimes patients may see "being held" (which they desire in a nonsexual way) as inherently tangled up with sexual contact. They may feel that sexual contact, or indeed any demand of the therapist, is a necessary price to pay for the seemingly saving, protective, and life-giving "holding." The transference in such cases is profound as is the patient's vulnerability.

* * *

In closing this chapter, it is important to note two crucial facts. First, while the ten scenarios described seem the most common avenues to therapists' sexual exploitation of their patients, they are by no means comprehensive. Second, while each scenario, in its general aspects, describes a large number of individual cases, each of the patients and therapists whom they describe experience this destructive event in his or her own way in the context of his or her unique life. Therapist-patient sexual intimacy is a deeply personal experience.

2

Attempts to Recognize, Define, and Address the Problem: Legal, Ethical, and Theoretical Conceptualizations

THE HISTORICAL ORIGIN AND RATIONALE FOR PROHIBITING THERAPIST-PATIENT SEXUAL INTIMACY

While therapist-patient sexual intimacy can appear in a variety of forms, as described in Chapter 1, it was nevertheless recognized as an abhorrent departure from acceptable practice—in any form—by the health care profession in its Hippocratic origins. The Hippocratic Oath makes a clear statement: "In every house where I come, I will enter only for the good of my patients, keeping myself far from all intentional ill-doing and all seduction, and especially from the pleasures of love with women and men" (*Dorland's Medical Dictionary* 1974, p. 175).

The reasons for this prohibition are many, and include three major issues. *First*, the prohibition recognizes the extreme vulnerability of the patient. Even the most assertive consumer-activist among us must still experience the trust and vulnerability of working with a "healer." When the concern is with our physical self, we allow the doctor to view the most private parts of our body. Even a routine examination customarily involves the patient disrobing. When surgery is involved, we allow doctors to cut into us, to remove parts of us, to see and touch parts of our inner workings that we ourselves have never seen or touched directly. In most major surgery, we as patients are not even conscious.

When the examination and treatment are of an emotional-psychological rather than physical nature, our vulnerability is just as great. We speak to therapists about our deepest secrets. We let them see us in our darkest and worst moments. In intense therapies, what a patient may blurt out is often as much (or more) a surprise to the patient as to the therapist. What emerges may evoke in the patient feelings of overwhelming shame, guilt, embarrassment, fear, anxiety, or confusion. A patient may frequently feel "out of control." Thus, in the same way that we allow a health care professional concerned with our physical health to examine and interact with our most private bodily parts, we allow a health care professional concerned with our emotional and psychological well-being to "see" our most private emotional and psychological aspects. Just as a careless move by a surgeon can have lethal consequences, careless words and other interventions by a psychotherapist can produce enormously destructive—sometimes lethal—consequences.

The exposure of our deepest, most private selves to psychotherapists is not the only aspect of vulnerability. There is also the fact that we customarily seek out health care professionals when we are hurting, when there is something wrong in our lives that is beyond our abilities to set right without help. We are acting out of pain and confusion, sometimes in desperation. In extreme cases, our fundamental ability to perceive, think, and remember clearly may be impaired. Those who suffer from Alzheimers Syndrome, drug overdoses, schizophrenic hallucinations and delusions, and strokes may be in a state of extreme vulnerability.

Still another aspect of vulnerability is the transference. Patients often come to invest their therapists with powers and characteristics that have less to do with the therapists than with the prior experiences and "psychology" of the patients. That this phenomenon occurs is neither unexpected nor harmful in and of itself. Indeed, the formation, analysis, and successful resolution of the transference are necessary processes in many therapeutic approaches. Nevertheless, anyone who has experienced this phenomenon is aware of the feelings of vulnerability that accompany it.

Because of such sources of vulnerability, the sexual intimacy that occurs between therapist and patient is very different from that which occurs in other situations. The multifaceted vulnerabilities of the patient create an enormous power differential, raising questions about the ability to give or withhold informed consent to participate in such intimacies. The resultant sexually intimate relationships therefore take on the aspects of and produce consequences similar to such phenomena as incest and rape. Such relationships are between one person who is seen as much more powerful and another person who is extremely vulnerable.

Aspects of the patient's vulnerability that form the basis for the prohibition against sexual involvement with a patient are summarized by Judd Marmor (1977, pp. 158–159), professor emeritus at the University of Southern California and a former president of the American Psychiatric Association:

> Such behavior is particularly reprehensible because of the special vulnerability of patients in this context. In many other relationships between a client and a professional, the client may be able to maintain a

certain amount of person reserve and still benefit from the relationship to a greater or lesser degree. In the psychotherapeutic relationship, however, a special emphasis is placed on the therapeutic necessity for the patient to set aside his or her customary defenses and to open himself or herself completely to the presumably benign and constructive influence of a therapist's professional skill. The implicit and explicit basis on which such total openness and trust is solicited is a solemn commitment that it will not be betrayed. Under such circumstances, a positive transference that leaves the patient uniquely vulnerable to the influence of the therapist usually develops. To exploit this iatrogenically induced vulnerability seems to me particularly reprehensible and unethical

The *second reason* for the prohibition focuses on the responsibilities of the therapist. Therapists view themselves as members of a profession. "Profession" in this sense means more than that the members receive money for what they do (as when the term is used to differentiate professional from amateur athletes). Nor is professional status in this sense conferred simply by virtue of training and ability to do a highly complicated task; such highly valuable blue-collar work as fixing an automobile engine or constructing an accurate watch would meet this criterion. When used in this manner, the term "professional" has historically referred to those who are willing to accept the honor, status, and other benefits of the designation in exchange for which they agree to place the welfare of those whom they serve foremost and to avoid any conflicting biases or confounding relationships.

This concept is one of great significance. An example of avoiding conflicting bias would be a surgeon performing two kidney operations in the same day. One involves a patient at the county hospital, a patient who has no funds. The other involves a millionaire who is a private patient of the physician. Any surgeon worthy of the term "professional" will not be more careless while performing the operation with one patient than with the other.

An example of avoiding a conflicting relationship is a lawyer who is asked to represent a client who is suing the lawyer's business partner. The lawyer will decline because she is aware that her relationship to her business partner will create an obstacle to her full and successful representation of the plaintiff.

Therapists who attempt to carry on sexual relationships with their therapy patients are engaging in an ethically indefensible dual relationship. They forfeit the unbiased objectivity and clarity necessary to render professional assessment and treatment. They allow their own wants and needs to sexual pleasure and intimacy to conflict with the patient's fundamental welfare.

A number of factors may lead therapists to jettison their intense commitment to the patient's best interests. Some therapists may have characterological flaws, and may feel little commitment to the welfare of patients to begin with. Perhaps they became therapists in order to make a lot of money, or to become famous and treat movie stars, or to engage in a voyeuristic exploration of the private lives of others, or to act out sadistic tendencies with vulnerable patients as victims. Others may, through lack of adequate training or psychological development, have inadequate control over their own impulses. Still others may be in a state of crisis themselves, may be what is termed "distressed or impaired therapists." Whatever the reasons, the abandonment of the commitment to the best interests of the patient is an abandonment of professional responsibilities and impairs or destroys altogether the ability to provide necessary diagnosis and treatment.

The *third reason* for the prohibition focuses on the harm that therapist-patient sexual intimacy inflicts upon patients. As Freud (whose work will be discussed later in this chapter) asserted and as the California study (Bouhoutsos et al. 1983) confirmed, when sexual intimacies begin, the therapy ends. Thus patients are deprived of the services they require and the therapist agreed to provide.

Beyond the abandonment of the therapeutic work, there are the numerous destructive sequelae to the sexual intimacy. The research reviewed in subsequent chapters has documented the profound, sometimes lethal, consequences.

Thus the prohibition against therapist-patient sexual intimacy, dating back at least 2,200 years, is based on at least three major areas: the vulnerabilities of the patient, the tasks and vulnerabilities of the provider, and the consequences for the patient. These three areas form the structure for Chapters 3, 4, and 5, which examine the more recent clinical and research findings.

THE MODERN AWAKENING TO THE PROBLEM

The prohibition against therapist-patient sexual intimacy, stated so eloquently in the Hippocratic Oath and so forcefully by Freud, has become a subject of widespread attention and concern in the last quarter of a century. Public interest has been reflected in a major narrative, *Betrayal* (Freeman and Roy 1976), subsequently made into a television movie; in large, front-page headlines (Brenneman 1978); in such popular columns as "Dear Abby" (Van Buren 1978), in the highly-rated television show *Sixty Minutes* (Glauber 1978); and in motion pictures with such major stars as Meryl Streep, Dudley Moore, and Roy Scheider (*Lovesick, Still of the Night*).

In the period spanning on the one hand the clear articulations of the prohibition by both Hippocrates and Freud and on the other hand the last 25 years, the issue lay relatively dormant. It did not appear explicitly in the ethics codes of the major mental health professions, went unmentioned in many texts, and was not a focus of clinical training.

Why the lack of explicit attention to this topic in the period immediately preceeding the last quarter century? The reason appears to be twofold.

First, the definitive proscriptions by Hippocrates and Freud appeared to be sufficient. It was simply assumed that therapist-patient sexual intimacy was such an egregious act on the part of the therapist that to include mention of it in, for instance, a textbook or ethical code would be entirely unnecessary. It would be like writing a manual for pilots on how to fly a plane and including the prohibition: "Do not crash the plane into the side of a mountain." The principle seems so obvious as to not need explicit mention.

Second, the topic makes so many mental health professionals nervous and uncomfortable that we tend to treat it with denial and "selective inattention," as described in Chapter 1. In the same way that the relatively recent massive attention paid by the public and the professions to the topics of rape, incest, and child abuse highlight the years of relative neglect due, at least in part, to our discomfort with those phenomena, so it was with the topic of therapist-patient sexual intimacy. The resistance to bringing the issue into our day-to-day awareness was enormous.

Specific examples of this denial and resistance are not hard to find. As late as 1977 a major article was published with a title characterizing therapist-patient sexual intimacy as the "problem with no name" (Davidson 1977).

Greenwald recounted his attempts to initate discussion of the subject at a meeting of the New York Psychological Association a quarter of a century ago: "I just raised the question . . . intending, as a clinical psychologist, that it be studied like any other phenomenon. And just for raising the question, some members circulated a petition that I should be expelled from the Psychological Association" (Shepard 1971, p.2).

About a decade later, Forer received approval from the Los Angeles County Psychological Association (in conjunction with the Los Angeles Society of Clinical Psychologists) to conduct a survey of the membership. On October 11, 1968, when he presented to the Board of Directors his findings showing a high rate of therapist-patient sexual intimacies, he was told that it was "not in the best interests of psychology to present it publicly" (Forer 1984). Although much later he was able to discuss his findings at general meetings of the association, he was able to disclose only "very restricted" aspects of his findings.

When Dahlberg was finally able to publish his paper on "Sexual Contact between Patient and Therapist" (1971), he wrote in the introduction: "I have had trouble getting this paper accepted by larger organizations where I had less, but still not inconsiderable influence. I was told that it was too controversial" (p. 34).

Even in recent questionnaire studies conducted by the authors of this book, some respondents are offended that the issue is being formally studied and either refuse to believe that any professionals would violate the fundamental prohibition against therapist-patient sexual intimacy or become angry at the researchers for studying the phenomenon.

If the dormancy of the issue has been due to the seemingly self-obvious nature of the prohibition and the discomfort of professionals in dealing with the subject, what accounts for the accumulating professional and public interest in the subject during the past quarter-century? Again, the reason appears to be twofold.

First, a very few therapists actually began to assert publicly that therapist-patient sexual intimacy could be a legitimate practice (McCartney 1966; Shepard 1971; Romeo 1978). (See Chapter 5 for a discussion of these assertions.) The result of these published attempts to legitimize sexual intimacies with patients had the opposite effect from what the authors apparently intended. It was as if the professions could tolerate some members violating the prohibition as long as they did so in relative privacy. Once the violators began to make public pronouncements, however, the professions were forced to respond. This type of situation is not new. Many groups seem adept at ignoring wrongs as long as they can claim to themselves and others that they are unaware, that they did not know what was happening (even if it is clear in hindsight that the evidence of the wrongs was all but unavoidable).

The minuscule number of advocates for legitimizing therapist-patient sexual intimacies thus helped force the professions into reexamining the reasons for the prohibition and acknowledging the need for explicit statements of that prohibition in ethical codes, textbooks, and so forth.

In addition, the briefs on behalf of therapist-patient sexual intimacy themselves served to reemphasize and clarify the soundness and necessity of the prohibition. For instance, Fritz Redlich, M.D., Professor of Psychiatry, Chair of Psychiatry, and Dean of the Medical School at Yale University, provide (1977, p. 150) the following analysis of Shepard's (1971) attempts to argue in favor of therapist-patient sexual intimacy:

> The hubris of this book really amazed me. Shepard recommends "mature" sexual relationships with patients, but every case in the book (verbatim accounts of patients' sexual relationships with other therapists) testifies to the breakdown of trust and regard and to the hostility and disappointment that follow the sexual involvement. The book also illustrates the psychopathological motivations of therapists who become thus involved. Such behavior satisfies the needs of the therapist, which are incompatible with good therapy, and not the legitimate needs of patients.

Second, patients began to press legal actions against therapists who violated the prohibition. The higher levels of the court system began affirming therapist-patient sexual intimacy as a sound basis for tort or malpractice actions with *Zipkin* v. *Freeman*, decided by the Missouri Supreme Court in 1968, and *Roy* v. *Hartogs,* decided by the New York Appellate Court in 1976. Traditionally, malpractice actions—particularly successful ones—have proved powerfully effective in getting the attention of mental health professionals. The juries have viewed with outrage therapists who have exploited vulnerable patients. The amount of the awards has varied from state to state. For example, Utah frequently makes awards in the low five figures; California for the same offense, has seen seven figures, such as $4.6 million (Shearer 1981). Even the most cynical therapists have been affected by this fact: both the size and the numbers of such awards have led insurance companies for psychiatrists, psychologists, and social workers to reduce substantially or eliminate altogether liability coverage relating to sexual intimacies with patients (Cummings and Sobel 1985). The figures are distressing: Insurance industry data suggest that 20 percent of all therapists will, some time during their careers, become sexually intimate with at least one of their patients (Los Angeles *Times*, February 14, 1976, p. 1).

It is important to note that it remains rare for therapist-patient sex cases to reach the courtroom. Insurance companies are generally reluctant to commit the time and expense necessary to undertake a trial, and they often attempt to reach a satisfactory out-of-court settlement. Most malpractice policies contain a provision that the therapist may be required to settle out of court at the discretion of the company. Frequently companies seek to protect the therapist (and themselves) from publicity that might lead to other patients filing suits against the same therapist by making the settlement contingent on the patient agreeing to forego filing a licensing complaint and/or making any public statements about the case or the size of the settlement. This limitation on the patient is sometimes extended to others involved in the case, such as attorneys and expert witnesses. This prohibition is open to question on the basis of its constitutionality (that is, freedom of speech), but this issue has not as yet been challenged in the courts.

The case of *Zipkin* v. *Freeman* has an interesting facet. Judge Seiler wrote the majority opinion of the Missouri Supreme Court, and concluded:

> The gravamen of the petition is that the defendant did not treat Mrs. Zipkin properly and as a result she was injured. He mishandled the transference phenomenon, which is a reaction the psychiatrists anticipate and which must be handled properly. (p. 761)

He discussed this point in more detail:

Once Dr. Freeman started to mishandle the transference phenomenon, with which he was plainly charged in the petition and which is overwhelmingly shown in the evidence, it was inevitable that trouble was ahead. It is pretty clear from the medical evidence that the damage would have been done to Mrs. Zipkin even if the trips outside the state were carefully chaperoned, the swimming done with suits on, and if there had been ballroom dancing instead of sexual relations. (p. 761)

The court thus recognizes and affirms the responsibility to handle properly the transference phenomenon as one of the major reasons for the prohibition against therapist-patient sexual involvement. Understanding of this point takes us back to Freud.

FREUD, TRANSFERENCE, AND COUNTERTRANSFERENCE

As Hippocrates had for an earlier period, Freud set forth in clear terms, with a solid theoretical basis, the prohibition of sexual relations with patients. A major reason for the prohibition involved the conceptualization of transference. In 1915 Freud differentiated the patient's transference as a clinical phenomenon from the nonclinical experience of "falling in love." He emphasized that the analyst "must recognize that the patient's falling in love is induced by the analytic situation and is not to be ascribed to the charms of his person, that he has no reason whatsoever therefore to be proud of such a 'conquest,' and it would be called outside analysis" (Freud 1963, p. 169). Freud believed this prohibition to be of fundamental importance for therapy and should serve the analyst as "a useful warning against any tendency to counter-transference which may be lurking in his own mind" (p. 169).

To engage in therapist-patient sex, Freud observed, means the destruction of the therapy. "If her advances were returned, it would be a great triumph for the patient, but a complete overthrow for the cure. . . . The love-relationship actually destroys the influence of the analytic treatment on the patient: a combination of the two would be an inconceivable thing" (p. 174).

So devastating were the consequences of sexual involvement with patients that Freud set forth prohibitions against kissing and other "preliminaries." He became quite concerned when Ferenczi, seeking to counteract parental unkindness by acting the part of the loving parent, began to become physically intimate with his patients. In a letter dated December 13, 1931, Freud wrote:

You have not made a secret of the fact that you kiss your patients and let them kiss you. . . . Now picture what will be the result of publishing your technique. . . . A number of independent thinkers in matters of technique will say to themselves: Why stop at a kiss? Certainly one gets further when one adopts "pawing" as well, which after all doesn't make a baby. And then bolder ones will come along who will go further, to peeping and showing—and soon we shall have accepted in the technique of analysis the whole repertoire of demi-viergerie and petting parties, resulting in an enormous increase of interest in psychoanalysis among both analysts and patients. The new adherent, however, will easily claim too much of this interest for himself; the younger of our colleagues will find it hard to stop at the point they originally intended, and God the Father Ferenczi, gazing at the lively scene he has created, will perhaps say to himself: Maybe after all I should have halted in my technique of motherly affection before the kiss (Jones 1957, pp. 163–164).

Freud's prohibition, as is true with so many sound notions, produced at least one unintended and unanticipated consequence. The traumatic and destructive aspects of sexual involvement with patients were stated so clearly by Freud that therapists began to be suspicious of any warm feelings toward patients. The evolution of the concept of countertransference, in particular, embodied this suspicion (see Pope, Keith-Spiegel, and Tabachnick 1986 for a review and discussion of this literature). As Thompson (1950, p. 107) described the situation:

Because of the stress on the unfortunate aspects of the analyst's involvement, the feeling grew that even a genuine objective feeling of friendliness on his part was to be suspected. As a result many of Freud's pupils became afraid to be simply human and show the ordinary friendliness and interest a therapist customarily feels for a patient. In many cases, out of a fear of showing counter-transference, the attitude of the analyst became stilted and unnatural.

This suspicion of feelings for the patient may have intensified the anxiety that is elicited by the topic of therapist-patient sexual involvement, and may still be a factor inhibiting the full recognition of this problem and our attempts to address it.

THE FORMAL STANDARDS

The few public statements endorsing therapist-patient sexual intimacy and the legal actions filed by patients served to begin mobilizing the mental health professions to address the issue in a more explicit manner. Research, which will be reviewed in subsequent chapters, was undertaken. The necessity of explicit, clear, and forceful prohibitions was recognized.

Beginning in the 1970s, each of the major mental health professions revised their ethical codes to include an explicit prohibition of sexual involvement with patients:

The necessary intensity of the therapeutic relationship may tend to activate sexual and other needs and fantasies on the part of both patient and therapist, while weakening the objectivity necessary for control. Sexual activity with a patient is unethical (American Psychiatric Association 1985).

Psychologists are continually cognizant of their own needs and of their potentially influential position vis-a-vis persons such as clients, students and subordinates. They avoid exploiting the trust and dependency of such persons. . . . Sexual intimacies with clients are unethical (American Psychological Association 1981).

The social worker should under no circumstances engage in sexual activities with clients (National Association of Social Workers 1980).

Sexual relationships between analyst and patient are antithetic to treatment and unacceptable under any circumstance. Any sexual activity with a patient constitutes a violation of this principle of ethics (American Psychoanalytic Association 1983)

A therapist will attempt to avoid relationships with clients which might impair professional judgment or increase the risks of exploiting clients. Examples of such relationships include: Treatment of family members, close friends, employees, or supervisees. Sexual activity with clients is unethical (American Association for Marriage and Family Therapy 1982).

Attempts were made to address this issue, then, by the courts (on the basis of suits filed by patients) and by the professional associations (primarily through explicit statements in their ethical codes). In addition, legislatures began to enable the government to take direct action against those professionals who violate the prohibition. In most cases the government (usually through the state boards that license therapists) initiates administrative hearings. All 50 states license psychiatrists and psychologists. Over half license social workers. A few license marriage and family therapists. The courts through such cases as *Morra* v. *State Board of Examiners* and *Cooper* v. *Board of Medical Examiners,* have affirmed the authority of licensing boards to revoke the licenses of therapists who violate the prohibition. About one-third of the states have passed legislation making therapist-patient sexual intimacy illegal, eliminating the need for expert testimony to establish the act as violating professional standards. In 1983 Wisconsin enacted legislation making sexual contact between therapist and patient a Class A misdemeanor (providing a sentence of up to nine months in jail and/or a $10,000 fine). The same legislation holds sexual intercourse between therapist and patient to be a class D felony (Wisconsin Act 434, 1983).

Finally, Masters and Johnson (1976), noting the many similarities between rape and therapist-patient sex, urged that therapists who exploit their power in order to have sexual relationships with patients should be charged with criminal rape. Redlich (1977) agreed in principle, but argued that a charge of statutory rape might be more appropriate. Other possible criminal charges would include fraud if the therapist were billing public assistance funds (such as Medicare) or private insurance companies for psychotherapeutic services when in fact he or she was substituting a sexual relationship for the purported therapy.

These recent efforts to address this major problem have unfortunately been far from a complete success, both in terms of preventing the phenomenon and in providing a redress of grievance for patients. For example, research findings have served as the basis of estimations that actions taken in all of these arenas (ethics committees, malpractice courts, licensing boards, and so on) amount to only about 4 percent of cases where sexual intimacy occurs, and only half of these are carried to completion (Bouhoutsos et al. 1983). The pressures against a patient filing a complaint are numerous, severe, and complex, and will be discussed in subsequent chapters, particularly Chapter 9. The reasons for the lack of action in response to all but a small proportion of the complaints that are filed are likewise numerous and complex. The most frequent reason given, whether by governmental agencies or professional associations, is lack of funding (Bouhoutsos 1984). For instance, a state licensing agency with limited funds spends an average of $7,000-$10,000 to investigate and adjudicate such cases, and much more if the therapist chooses to engage in delaying tactics and full appeals (Vinson 1984). The prospects for addressing this phenomenon more effectively, particularly in terms of prevention, are discussed in Chapter 12.

3

Therapists
at Risk

What kind of psychotherapists are at risk for becoming sexually involved with their patients? Information about such therapists has been difficult to obtain. Patients who file complaints against these therapists frequently must undergo psychological evaluations, but the therapists who have damaged them are usually not subject to such evaluations. Were such psychological studies possible, we could construct a more accurate typology of therapists who become sexually involved with patients. Such studies might also suggest ways in which such therapists could be helped if, indeed, they can be helped.

Through anonymous self-report studies we have gathered some information about the general class of such therapists: their number, demographic characteristics, and pattern of erotic and nonerotic activity with patients. Table 2 summarizes the rates of therapist-patient sex obtained by the studies conducted to date.

Differences due to such factors as the dates of the studies, geographic locales, and the selection criteria prohibit firm conclusions about possible differences among the professions. A research project that studies all of these professions (thus minimizing the differences in selection criteria, dates of sampling, and such) is needed.

Data collected from a study of marriage and family counselors are now being analyzed. When that is completed, an overview of sexual involvement with patients on the part of all of the mental health disciplines will be available.

From the data available, therapists tend to be from 12 to 16 years older than their female patients with whom they are involved (Butler 1975). They tend to be well established in practice; some have been leaders in the field. Several attempts have been made to understand the dynamics of patient-therapist involvement on the part of the therapist. Some analysts postulate

TABLE 2.   Studies of Therapist-Patient Sexual Intimacy Frequencies

Ref. No.	Pub. Date	Profession	Location	Return Rate (percent)	Males	Females
1	1968	Psychologists	Los Angeles County	70	13.7	0
2	1973	Psychiatrists	Los Angeles County	46	10.0	n/a
3	1976	Psychiatrists	California & New York	33	n/a	0
4	1977	Psychologists	National	70	12.1	2.6
5	1979	Psychologists	National	48	12.0	3.0
6	1985	Social Workers	National	54	3.8	0
7	1986	Psychiatrists	National	26	7.1	3.1
8	1986	Psychologists	National	59	9.4	2.5

Reference Key:
1 Forer [1980]
2 Kardener, Fuller, and Mensh
3 Perry
4 Holroyd and Brodsky
5 Pope, Levenson, and Schover
6 Gechtman and Bouhoutsos
7 Gartrell, Herman, Olarte, Feldstein, and Localio
8 Pope, Keith-Spiegel, and Tabachnick

an underlying hostility on the part of the male therapists against their mothers, and their need to have patients mother them (S. Smith 1981). When the patients refuse to continue this mothering and start to demand more attention, love, or commitment from the therapist the involvement is no longer desirable. The therapist withdraws, and the patient feels abandoned, betrayed, and used. The patient stops paying for "treatment" and that is when the lawsuit or the ethics complaint is filed.

Research efforts were made to obtain empirical information about such therapists. Advertisements were placed on local bulletin boards and in newspapers. Resultant dissertations (Butler 1975; D'Addario 1977) revealed that 60 percent of the erotic therapists saw themselves as father figures; 70 percent recognized that they were in a more dominant role than their patients; 55 percent were frightened of intimacy; and 95 percent reported fear and guilt over what happened. Only 40 percent sought help from a friend or colleague. Some 45 percent rationalized their behavior by indicating that they became sexually involved with their patients because of the expressed need of those patients. Butler pointed out that the typical psychotherapist has been taught that countertransference feelings are to be avoided in the therapeutic situation. She postulated that since there is little opportunity for those feelings to find social or professional expression, they are often repressed as signs of emotional inadequacy—feelings that should be recognized and analyzed are suppressed and denied. Consequently, the therapist projects onto the patient his or her own unresolved countertransference.

The neglect of sexual countertransference in the training of psychotherapists brings us to the more general topic of sexual attraction to patients. Such attraction, in any given instance, may or may not involve countertransferential elements. Therapists' sexual attraction to their patients, though generally neglected as a topic of research, seems to be a widespread phenomenon. Pope, Keith-Spiegel, and Tabachnik (1986), in a national survey of psychologists, found that the vast majority (87 percent) reported having experienced sexual attraction to their patients. The attraction seems to be more common among male (95 percent) than female (76 percent) therapists, but was acknowledged by a very large percentage (88 percent) of younger female psychologists.

The lack of attention to this topic in training programs and research studies is quite understandable in light of the acute discomfort it seems to cause for the individual practitioner. Many (63 percent) reported feeling guilty, anxious, or confused about this sexual attraction to their patients.

What were the characteristics of the patients to whom the therapists were attracted? The list was long, but among the most frequently mentioned attributes were physical attractiveness, positive mental traits (intelligent, articulate), sexual features (sexual ideal, sexy), and vulnerability (needy, child-like, sensitive, fragile). Almost all the characteristics were mentioned with roughly equal frequencies by male and female psychologists except for two. "Physical attractiveness" was much more often mentioned by male than by female psychologists; "successful" was mentioned far more often by female than male psychologists. This gender difference seems to reflect more general trends within our culture. The attraction was exclusively to clients of the opposite sex for 85 percent of the male and 66 percent of the female psychologists. The sexual attraction was to both male and female clients for 14 percent of the male and 31 percent of the female psychologists. The attraction was exclusively to clients of the same sex for 0.6 percent of the male and 3 percent of the female therapists.

Only 7 percent acted on these feelings (that is, engaged in sexual intimacies with patients), but 18 percent considered doing so. All of those who reported attraction to patients but who did not become sexually involved were asked why they refrained from the involvement. Many provided more than one reason, and 1,091 responses were the result. Among the most frequent categories of response were statements that therapist-patient sexual intimacy is: (1) unethical, (2) countertherapeutic or exploitive, (3) an unprofessional practice, and (4) against the therapist's personal values. Such statements appear to reflect a view beyond narrow self-interest. They express commitment to the standards of the profession, a regard for the patient's well-being, and personal values in tune with professional values.

Less often cited as reasons for refraining from sexual contact with patients were: (5) being in a committed relationship with someone else, (6) fear of censure or loss of reputation, (7) damage to the therapist, (8) fear of retaliation by the patient, and (9) awareness that such behavior is illegal.

These latter, less frequently cited reasons appear to focus on what is best for the therapist (particularly in terms of avoiding negative effects for the therapist).

It is worth noting here that the responses to this questionnaire, while anonymous, may be prone to an unspecifiable amount of distortion in the attribution of causes for refraining from sex with patients. Some respondents may have been motivated to provide what they viewed as more personally or socially acceptable answers. The validity of this research in this particular area will await further investigation. At present, however, these data constitute the only systematically gathered, empirically derived information we have on this subject, and thus may be the best basis for inferences.

These data suggest that for many—but by no means all—therapists, the external systems of restraint and prohibition may be relatively ineffective in preventing therapist-patient sexual involvement. These findings point us in two directions: (1) paying more attention to the personal and professional values of the candidate as one criterion for admission to therapy training programs, and (2) examining more closely the resources that training programs can provide that will enhance these values and will better equip therapists to refrain from sexual involvement with patients.

In terms of the training programs themselves, there are few that adequately address issues relating to the exploration of fantasies about and sexual feelings for patients. About half of the psychologists did not receive any guidance or training in such issues at all, and only 9 percent reported that their training and supervision were adequate.

Pope, Keith-Spiegel, and Tabachnik (1986) provide criteria of educational programs that could effectively address issues related to sexual attraction to and sexual involvement with patients. At the very least we can say that the temptation of a sexual relationship with a vulnerable, adoring patient needs more attention than a brief mention during a review of the Hippocratic Oath or a casual comment during an ethics course.

A crucial point is that sexual attraction to patients and sexual involvement with patients, while related in some cases, are nevertheless distinct issues. Therapists and therapists-in-training may feel so guilty about being attracted to a patient because they feel it is "as if" they were already or were about to become sexually intimate with the patient. However, the phenomenon of sexual attraction to patients appears to be (statistically) normal, and may be a completely natural part of the therapist's reaction to some patients. In some cases it may represent countertransference; in other cases it may represent an undistorted human reaction to another person; but in all cases the urge to become sexually involved must be resisted. In virtually all cases such feelings, if they are handled in an open, sensitive, and professional manner, can constitute a useful therapeutic resource.

Therapy training programs not only generally fail to address the issues of therapist attraction to and involvement with patients, but also—when they do address these issues—generally fail to do so in an effective manner. That is to say, the training program curricula dealing with these issues, as presently constituted, do not seem to be effective in enabling therapists to resist the impulse to engage in sexual relations with a patient. Gechtman and Bouhoutsos (1985), for example, in a national study of social workers, found that social workers who had graduated from training programs that addressed these issues had the same rate of sexual involvement with patients as those who graduated from training programs that ignored the issues.

Why the ineffectiveness of such programs, at least among social work schools? Several hypotheses are possible: the courses offered are inadequate, the therapists are so distressed by conditions in their lives that their own needs supercede their ethical judgment, or the therapists have characterological problems that prevent didactic or therapeutic intervention. We will consider each of these possibilities.

THE POORLY TRAINED PSYCHOTHERAPIST

The most usual explanation offered for sexual involvement on the part of a therapist with a patient is that he or she "did not know any better." However, we are aware that many senior, well-established mental health professionals have been involved with their patients, and in some instances even married them (Bouhoutsos, 1984). The male psychotherapists involved with female patients have tended to be in their forties and fifties with a long history of training and experience. Despite this evidence that most therapists do indeed "know better," there are some common misconceptions that could influence their decision to become involved sexually with a patient, and that merit mentioning here.

The first misconception is that sexual involvement with a patient is acceptable if it occurs outside the therapeutic session. It is not uncommon for a therapist to tell a patient that it is unethical to have sexual relations during the therapeutic hour, but that they should meet in the evening, in her or his home or a motel. This would appear to be the unlikeliest of misconceptions were it not for the wording of ethics codes, which sometimes state prohibitions against therapist/patient sex "during therapy." Some therapists misinterpret this admittedly awkward wording to mean "during each therapeutic session." There have been no instances of this defense being used successfully in ethics hearings, licensing actions, or civil court as far as we know.

The second misconception is that only sexual involvement that occurs prior to the termination of therapy is illegal and/or unethical. Frequently one hears this as a defense in both ethics and administrative law hearings. Usually therapy has been terminated by the therapist in order to begin a sexual relationship with the patient. A recent study of psychology licensing boards and state psychological associations (Gottlieb, Sell, and Schoenfeld 1985) surveyed the number of instances therapists used therapy termination as a defense. Quite a number did so but in no instance was the individual cleared on that basis. On the other hand, no state had a regulation spelling out a particular time limit when a therapeutic relationship could end and a social/sexual relationship begin. The study calls for a clear statement in ethics, administrative, and civil codes that a sexual relationship is never possible between a therapist and a client since this appears to be a currently unstated policy. The American Psychological Association Ethics Committee made such a formal statement in June 1986.

The third misconception is that sexual involvement with a patient is acceptable if the patient initiates it. This contention frequently is brought up by attorneys but rarely by therapists as a defense. It has no merit. *The responsibility for the relationship always rests with the therapist no matter what the behavior of the patient.* Whether or not the patient was seductive is of no concern except as grist for the therapeutic mill.

The fourth misconception is that if one's professor or supervisor or colleague was involved with a patient without being disciplined, one can also indulge with impunity. This is usually an unstated misperception and rarely adduced in any type of hearing. However, it does frequently determine the attitude about sexual relations with patients taken by the mental health professional establishing a practice. Pope, Levenson, and Schover (1979) found that students engaging in erotic activity with professors was significantly correlated with later sexual contact with clients (at least for women). It is not unusual to find dynasties of therapists who become sexually involved with their patients who have been taught by a professor who habitually became involved with students. Rather than group practices counteracting such tendencies, it is sometimes the case that all of the members of the group participate.

These four misconceptions need attention in the educational programs preparing psychotherapists for practice. Those medical schools and other graduate programs that do not attend to these matters are providing inadequate training for their students and share in the responsibility for damaging patients.

THE DISTRESSED PSYCHOTHERAPIST

Historically, mental health professionals have been reluctant to view themselves as troubled human beings. Medicine's homily, "doctors make the worst patients," certainly includes psychiatrists, psychologists, social workers, and family therapists. Many psychotherapeutic disciplines have built into their educational process an obligatory "training analysis," and this has allowed students to mask their treatment for emotional problems under the guise of a learning experience in preparation for their future professions. Faced with situations beyond their coping capabilities, many professionals find it difficult to acknowledge their fallibility. When they do, they frequently find that they have no place to turn. Most hesitate to reveal their difficulties to their families, which may be part of the problem and provide little support. Even when these distressed therapists turn to colleagues, as a surprising 57 percent of psychologists in California revealed they had done in cases of sexual involvement with clients (Bouhoutsos et al. 1983), it is likely that those colleagues to whom they turned were ill equipped to deal with such confidences and most likely minimized the problem or "swept the instance under the rug."

Even more difficult are such problems when therapists themselves fail to recognize the severity of their disturbances. Often their colleagues become aware of their distress either through shared patients or through clinical sensitivity to aberrant behavior. Some ethics codes (American Psychological Association 1981) require that if a member of a professional association notices a breach of ethics has been committed, he or she should speak to the offender before taking formal action. But how does one tell one's colleagues that they are drinking too much, that they are exhibiting severe attentional or memory disturbances, or that their judgment is faulty and that they should seek help?

One deterrent to addressing these problems directly with a colleague is that one is afraid to be seen as an adversary rather than a concerned colleague. Professional associations are not usually helpful in this regard. Ethics committees do not usually intervene until after there is a complaint, and they are usually viewed as educative or even punitive rather than rehabilitative. Even when the impaired psychologist exhibits insight and motivation there is still a lack of identified resource people who can provide the specialized information necessary in cases of sexual involvement with clients.

The reluctance and inability of the professions to deal with colleagues in distress has resulted in tragedy in many instances. As a hypothetical example, a psychotherapist is noticeably agitated, quarrelsome, and depressed on occasion. Only later do colleagues realize that his uncharacteristic behavior signals a need for help. For a long period of time, he is treated with impatience and irritation when he behaves irrationally at meetings. Subsequent acting-out behavior with patients is similarly overlooked until there is an explosion of violence in which the man kills a patient, his family, and himself. A psychological autopsy reveals that there had been innumerable clues that pointed to increasing emotional disorder, any of which, if followed up, could have averted the tragedy. Sensitivity to his distress and resources for referral are significantly absent.

The medical profession was the first to establish a program for helping impaired colleagues (R. Smith 1980). However, in 1971 a survey of state medical societies indicated that only seven states provided a committee to oversee such a program and only two states had statutes that provided for disciplinary and therapeutic intervention. These two states, Florida and Texas, had created a "sick doctor" statute that permitted action before injury to patients. The American Medical Association (AMA) released a statement in 1972 maintaining that physicians had an ethical responsibility to recognize and report impairment in colleagues (AMA, Council on Mental Health 1973), and in 1974 a model act was drafted that permitted licensing boards to give rehabilitative and therapeutic care to medical practitioners prior to actual patient injury. By 1982, 101 citations were reported in a computer search and all 50 state medical societies had impaired physician committees. Self-help groups, similar to Alcoholics Anonymous, have been helpful for many types of problems, and are available for most professionals (for example, International Lawyers in Alcoholics Anonymous [Laliotis and Grayson 1985]). Psychologists have been somewhat slower than other professional groups to recognize the problems of impaired colleagues. A study (Abell and Strong 1983) that compared law, medicine, psychology, dentistry, nursing, and social work found that even in responding to a questionnaire about rehabilitation of impaired members, state psychological associations responded less frequently. Nursing had the highest rate of response. Medicine indicated the greatest interest in rehabilitation of distressed colleagues, psychology the least.

The California State Psychological Association has been attempting to establish a program for distressed psychologists for approximately five years. Described as the having "made the most progress in program development" of all the states (Laliotis and Grayson 1985), the program is partially in place but faces dilemmas and difficulties that appear to defy solution.

Only the self-referred cases offer possibility of intervention without excessive complication, and therapist-patient sexual involvement does not ordinarily fall within this category. Yet it seems clear that many of those therapists who become sexually involved with their patients are distressed. Is there evidence that therapists are aware of their own distress?

A recent study of all licensed psychologists in California attempted to assess the degree of adherence to the Standards of Providers of Psychological Services by the members of the profession (Bouhoutsos 1983). Questionnaires were sent to the approximately 5,500 licensees and 65 percent responded; Part II of the study, which contained an item on distress, was sent to a random sample (1,200 of the 5,500). They were asked to complete an additional section and 50 percent complied. The questionnaire did not seek identifying data and the respondents were assured of anonymity. The question directed toward distress read: "During the past year, have you experienced any of the following problems that may have diminished your ability to maintain effective professional practice?" In response, 523 (90 percent) answered no; 35 (6 percent) answered yes; 23 (4 percent) gave no response. The yes responses were made to the following categories:

Alcohol abuse: 6 (1 percent)
Compulsive gambling: 0
Major mental illness: 6 (1 percent)
Other substance abuse: 3 (0.5 percent)
Major physical illness or disability: 9 (1.5 percent)
Grief over loss or separation from loved one: 23 (4 percent)
Other: 14 (2 percent)

The study did not include a specific item on sexual intimacy with patients. However, since 90 percent of those therapists sexually involved with patients reported feeling vulnerable, needy, or lonely when the sexual contact occurred and many were separated, divorced, or unhappily married, it is possible that those 4 percent who indicate problems in their relationships might have contained a substantial number who were involved sexually with patients. Thus there would appear to be a pool of individuals who might benefit from a Distressed Therapist program that offers assistance in times of crisis. Difficulty arises when there is need to differentiate the distressed therapist from the exploitive therapist. The state of the art in psychological assessment is such that we can no more acurately predict recidivism in the area of sexual acting out than in criminal behavior.

One approach has been to design a model that encompasses both the distressed and the distressing psychotherapist, the former in need of assistance, the latter needing containment.

Currently, the possibility of rehabilitating mental health professionals who have been sexually involved with their patients is a difficult problem for both professional organizations and licensing boards. When ethics committees or licensing boards stipulate that such psychologists go into therapy and/or be supervised by senior psychologists, there is generally no provision, or capability, for monitoring that person. Since the early literature shows that 80 percent of those psychologists involved sexually with their patients act out with more than one person (Holroyd and Brodsky 1977), it is with understandable reluctance that the committees and boards, charged with protecting the public welfare, allow these psychologists to return to practice.

Monitoring is almost impossible, since if the therapist is aware of the monitoring he or she can act out away from the office (and usually does). Limiting practices to all one gender is also not very feasible. First, loss of one-third to one-half a patient load presents an economic consideration taken into account by judges. Second, therapists may not confine their sexual acting out to one gender. Third, the cost of monitoring is usually prohibitive.

A program that offers a continuum from the distressed therapist to the rigorous containment approach is, of course, optimal. Unfortunately, we have not as yet solved the problems of selection and enforcement, among others. One model (devised by Bouhoutsos for use by the California State Psychological Association) allocates responsibility for such program to three bodies: the Distressed Psychologist program, the Ethics Committee, and the State Licensing Board. There are three levels:

Level I: Self-referred. An individual seeks support from the system for a personal problem. This type of request is rarely received by a state professional association ethics committee and practically never by a licensing board. However, this is the type of case that is best served by a Distressed Therapist program. An arms' length relationship is necessary between this program and enforcement bodies such as professional ethics committees and/or licensing boards.

The Distressed Therapist program is set up under the aegis of a professional organization or, preferably, organizations, since all therapists appear to suffer from the same types of problems and sometimes prefer to consult another discipline.

One difficulty in establishing such programs has been suspicion on the part of the membership of professional organizations that confidentiality might not be sufficiently protected. If therapists are to feel comfortable in using this service, it is imperative that rigorous standards of confidentiality be maintained. Locked files, purged when cases are completed, are a necessity. Statistics about participation are desirable, but care should be taken to omit any type of identifying data.

Information about the distressed program should be widely distributed through newsletters and personal communications to all licensed professionals in the disciplines, stressing confidentiality and availability. If possible, an 800 number should be provided and anonymous inquiries encouraged.

A panel of specifically trained senior professionals should be available for referral. Existing national self-help organizations such as Physicians Helping Physicians or Psychologists Helping Psychologists should be included as resources. The self-help group model has been found more effective in certain addiction and behavior problems than other types of therapy.

Frequently licensing boards are under legal constraints that do not allow them to refer to professional associations or to individuals. However, complaints that do not support disciplinary actions are frequently forwarded to ethics committees and if these complaints are seen by those committees as not involving ethical violations, referral to the Distressed Therapist program is in order.

Level II: Self-referred or other-referred cases involving alcohol or drug use that might result or have resulted in poor service to patients. This level could also include therapists who have had sexual relations with patients. Self-referrals are not frequent in this category. Most referrals in this category are received from Ethics, Peer Review, Standards, or other Quality of Care committees, or a Licensing Board. The therapist may have been referred as part of a stipulation; that is, he or she would have agreed to undertake a particular course of action in return for retaining membership in an organization or a license to practice. Such action frequently requires a course of therapy and/or supervision. The committee or licensing board makes the individual aware of the professional organization program, as well as others, which are available. Those senior professionals on the Distressed Therapist panel who provide therapy and/or supervision are responsible for providing regular reports to the referral source about the progress made and recommendations as to the continuance of membership or licensure. Report is made to the licensing board regarding attendance and successful completion of the program. A waiver of confidentiality is necessary in these cases. Fees are paid by the therapist in the program.

Level III: Referrals from licensing boards only. Referral is made by the licensing board when therapy and supervision are mandatory conditions of reinstatement. Fees are paid by the probationer. The Distressed Psychologist panel names (among others) are supplied to the therapist. In the case of the licensing board, monitoring is done by the probation officer, if the therapist is still on probation. Since probation reports are part of the public domain there is no confidentiality. The court can request evidence of rehabilitation. The treating therapist who is called upon to provide such evidence must be scrupulouly objective. Recent research has addressed the question of bias when the reporter comments on his or her own activity, whether as actor or consultant (Holroyd and Bouhoutsos 1985).

THE THERAPIST WITH CHARACTEROLOGICAL PROBLEMS

On the opposite end of the continuum from the distressed therapist is the individual with characterological problems who tends toward repetition of sexual involvement. Early research indicated that if a therapist had sex with one patient, in 80 percent of the cases it recurred with other patients

(Holroyd and Brodsky 1977). A recent study (Pope, Keith-Spiegel, and Tabachnik 1986) found that while 86 percent of those who became sexually intimate with patients did so once or twice, 10 percent did so between three and ten times, and one psychologist, a woman, reported a frequency of over ten times. Another source reported a therapist, a man, who had been involved with as many as 100 patients (Siegel 1983). Because so few empirical data are available on the personalities of those therapists sexually involved with their patients, we can only speculate that these therapists who become sexually involved with patients repetitively might have characterological problems in contrast to being "distressed." Legal systems have used the concept of recidivism to determine punishment and psychologists have identified past behavior as the most viable criterion on which to predict dangerousness (Shah 1980). Some of the vignettes presented in Chapter 1, for instance "Svengali" and "Rape," illustrate the degree to which the characterological styles of the therapist contribute to therapist-patient sexual involvement.

DISCUSSION

Therapists may display characterologically based destructive styles in a variety of forms. They may be sadistic, exploitive, or masochistic. They may seek to create massive dependency on the part of the patient, or they may develop substantial dependency on the patient. They may be power-hungry, abusive, impulsive, or coldly hostile. All, however, are in need of assistance, both professional and collegial. They are also in need of external monitoring and restraint—to prevent them from causing deep, lasting, and sometimes fatal harm to their patients—which they are unable to supply by and for themselves.

Members of the mental health professions who are experiencing burn-out, mid-life crisis, family problems, or romantic difficulties deserve help in recognizing their own vulnerabilities and seeking professional help. The fact that 57 percent of those sexually involved with patients had turned to colleagues (Bouhoutsos et al. 1983) and that these colleagues tended to be biased (Holroyd and Bouhoutsos 1985) suggests, however, that care be taken to provide assistance by an expert in the area of patient-therapist sexual involvement. If one becomes aware that a colleague is experiencing such distress, it is helpful to be aware of resource people in the community and to call upon them for assistance in helping that colleague. Readings on the topic can be helpful in understanding the problem and its consequences.

Those therapists who feel uncomfortable with patients they view as "seductive" might also seek out a colleague with experience in the area of patient-therapist intimacy. There should be no stigma attached to peer review, and case discussions can be eminently helpful in avoiding damaging entanglements. The discussion of sexuality with a patient can be titillating, and certainly arousing, and it is important to recognize that such arousal is not unusual. Perhaps the most difficult trap to avoid is the feeling that one is indispensable, that only through personal intervention can one provide a patient with the feeling that he or she is lovable, desirable, and worthwhile. Rescuers in the helping professions are particularly prone to encourage attenuated dependency on the therapist and to discourage social networks, a reversal of the healing process (see Chapter 8). Therapy that continues through many years without concern for creating independence merits observation and monitoring.

Exploitive and power-hungry therapists represent a more difficult problem. It is unlikely that any intervention now known can provide a solution. More will be said about this group in Chapters 10 and 12 on the legal and ethical systems.

4

Vulnerabilities
of Patients

What kind of patients become sexually involved with their therapists? Patients who enter the office of a therapist for the first time are usually filled with a mix of hope, anticipation, fear, and anxiety. Most have a great deal of pain, enough to make them willing to endure the fear and anxiety and to pay for the privilege of undergoing the further pain of self-exploration and confrontation. Because of the promise of relief, a patient shares hidden thoughts, fantasies, and emotions and grows to trust the therapist, who promises confidentiality, concern, and help in return for that trust. Discussion of the necessity of a trusting relationship is customarily a part of therapy, and therapists frequently emphasize complete trust as a requisite for progress in the therapeutic process (Marmor 1972b). On the assumption that this trust will not be betrayed, the patient is encouraged to set aside customary defenses and open up to the therapist's probing. Interactions during therapy are intimate and personal and encourage warmth and closeness.

Also a part of therapy is the tacit recognition of the unequal power distribution between therapist and patient. This power differential, which favors the therapist, may create unrealistic feelings of superiority (Marmor 1953). The neediness of the patient, the discomfort that has necessitated the search for surcease, the mythic or actual knowledge with which the therapist is endowed, and the trappings of the office purvey this power differential and color the therapeutic interchange.

A safeguard against unbridled use of power in the therapeutic process is the "frame of therapy" that limits the boundaries of the relationship and offers security for the participants. This frame establishes safe boundaries (A.A. Stone 1983) within which the patient assumes there will be confidentiality, freedom from conflicts of interest, and unequivocal concern on the part of the therapist for his or her welfare as a consumer. These elements of therapy—trust, power, and framing—are the crucial areas that are violated when the therapeutic relationship is sexualized.

The research has tended to focus on therapeutic dyads in which the therapist is male and patient is female (Bouhoutsos et al. 1983). Therefore, much of the following discussion will refer to female patients and their response to the actions of male therapists. It is extremely important to keep in mind that therapist-patient sexual intimacy is by no means limited to such patterns. The research clearly shows that sexual intimacy occurs also in cases where both individuals are female, where both individuals are male, and where the therapist is female and the patient is male. Nor is therapist-patient sex limited to dyadic situations. For example, some therapists involve their patients in group sex.

Although several dissertations have explored the characteristics of female patients who have become involved with male therapists, and some familiar adjectives are repeated in the literature, we still lack definitive descriptors that would assist us in identifying women at risk for such involvements. Three categories of patients do emerge, however, from the clinical experience of the authors that merit discussion:

1. The low-risk group: Highly stressed patients who have no history of prior hospitalization, are normally high functioning, come from a stable family background, and who have had previous long-term fulfilling intimate emotional and sexual relationships,

2. The middle-risk group: Patients who give a history of prior relationship problems, appear to be somewhat dependent and needy, and may fall into the personality disorder category,

3. The high-risk group: Patients who have a history of previous hospitalizations, suicide attempts, major psychiatric illnesses, and drug or alcohol addiction problems.

From an examination of these three categories, it is understandable why the literature contains disparate views of patients who become sexually involved with their therapists. The variability of the patients is similar to that found among the therapists described in Chapter 3 and categorization in either instance is at best tentative and descriptive.

THE LOW-RISK GROUP

Robertiello (1975) describes a sample of patients sexually involved with their therapists who appear to fit the low-risk criterion. He sees them as well within the norm, not especially "sick," suggestible, masochistic, "prone to symbiosis," nor schizophrenic or even borderline. He identifies their problems as neurotic conflicts, he views these women as possessing many strengths including intelligence, ego strength, and the ability to cope quite effectively with reality. Seven of the eight patients he interviewed had finished college; all held jobs. Several of them were married and had children. He does not see them as particularly masochistic. He summed up his findings by pointing out that these women were people not different from any "of us"; in fact, several were remarkably gifted and talented. "What happened to them could have happened to any one of our patients and perhaps even to any one of us" (p. 6).

A frequent precursor for a patient of the low-risk category to enter therapy is a traumatic occurrence in a relationship. If that patient chooses a therapist who has been sexually involved with other patients, and if this patient is sufficiently stressed, she may be at increased risk. The following fictional examples illustrate the low-risk category.

Example 1. Sandy was an attractive, bright, well-functioning young professional involved for a number of years in a satisfying relationship with a man she loved. When he became enamored with another woman, Sandy became deeply depressed. A friend referred her to a well-established psychotherapist, and Sandy saw him approximately three times. Most of her time in his office was spent in tears over her loss. Her weeping was also for her loss of self-esteem over the rejection. During the third session, the therapist put his arms around her to comfort her, then began to kiss her. She was immobilized and could not fend off his insistent disrobing and he penetrated her. When he was satisfied she stumbled from the office, got into her car, and began driving erratically. She sped along a curved mountain road, seriously considering driving over the cliff and ending her initial pain, which now was overlaid with guilt, disgust, hatred, and anger.

Example 2. John and Mary had been married for seven years and had one five-year-old child, but the marriage was not faring well. John enjoyed mountain climbing and frequently went away on weekends with his friends. Mary was enrolled in college and spent a great deal of her time studying for her degree. The child was experiencing some school difficulties and needed help with school work. John felt that the house was neglected. The washing and cleaning were not being done, and he was acutely uncomfortable with the deteriorating standards. He was increasingly critical of Mary and finally both of them decided that they needed some help with the marriage.

The couple went to a marriage counselor who began seeing them together. Soon she requested to see them separately. To each of them she said the other was unsuitable as a marriage partner. She began hugging, kissing, and fondling the wife. Although the wife grew increasingly uncomfortable as the hugs turned into erotic caresses, she felt sufficiently alienated from her husband not to share this information with him. The therapist suggested to the husband that he divorce his wife since the relationship appeared hopeless.

As the husband moved further away emotionally, the therapist moved closer to the wife and engaged in a number of sexual activities with her. As the wife's demands on the therapist became more insistent, she lost interest and became involved with another patient. The wife was left without her husband, with a child who had been neglected and was consequently experiencing difficulties in school, with little money, since the bill for therapy had continued to appear monthly, and with feelings of betrayal, guilt, and self-hate.

THE MIDDLE-RISK GROUP

The patient population described most frequently in the literature appears to fall within this middle-risk group. Theories about the etiology of the "at risk" factor are varied. Several feminist authors have underlined the culpability of society and of most psychotherapists for perpetuating a stereotype of femininity. Chesler (1972) identified certain characteristics that she defined as traditionally feminine: other-directedness, little self-regard, and little acceptance of their own aggression. D'Addario (1977) stated that these characteristics are considered normal and healthy in women from the perspective of society but emphasized that they contribute to women's psychopathology and perpetuate feminine stereotypes. She quotes an earlier study (Broverman et al. 1970) in which male and female psychologists expect women to be more passive and dependent than men, while recognizing that these traits are not conducive to optimal functioning.

Chesler (1972) interviewed eleven women, ten of whom had had sex with their therapists. She describes them as "unambivalent" about their femininity. All were economically limited, intellectually insecure, conventionally and "frantically" attractive, sexually fearful on the one hand and sexually compulsive on the other. "They were paralyzed by real and feared loneliness and self-contempt" (p. 149). All of them blamed themselves for their "mistreatment" by men. The ages of the women ranged from 22 to 45. Their therapists were an average of 15 years older. Four women were separated or divorced, four were married, three were single. Many described their sexual involvement with the therapist as being gradual. In another study (Bouhoutsos et al. 1983) many of the women did not realize at first that there was anything amiss. Although at times they questioned the holding, fondling, kissing, and eventual intercourse which took place, if the therapist whom they trusted assured them it was part of therapy or for their own good, most believed and complied. Those who objected were frequently threatened with termination of therapy and were so needy and so bound to the therapeutic lifeline that they yielded to the power of the therapist and acquiesced. Once sex began and the therapeutic frame was violated, the decline of the process was inevitable.

Belote (1974) examined the traits of high femininity described by Chesler—other-directedness, low self-regard, low acceptance of aggression and masochism—to verify if they were characteristic of women who were at risk for sexual involvement with their therapists. The majority of Belote's sample of women were young, above average in attractiveness, intelligent, unmarried and living alone, had some college education, and were unemployed. Depression was the most prevalent presenting problem but a variety of other problems were noted: anxiety attacks, feelings of isolation, preoccupation with suicide, marital conflicts, and phobias. This was a first therapy experience for 15 of the 25 women and most felt that they had no other alternative and could not have handled their problems without therapeutic assistance. Three of the women were virgins and had had no sexual experience at all prior to entering therapy. Thirteen had never experienced orgasm and an additional five had only a few. Thus a total of 18 out of 25 women had orgasmic difficulties. However, none of women gave sexual dysfunction as the presenting problem. Many of the women reported feeling that their fathers were sexually attracted to them during their puberty and felt that their mothers were jealous of them. Five women had been raped once or twice prior to commencing therapy, two by family members. Three of the women had been prostitutes. Five of the women had been propositioned by a previous therapist. The majority of the women reported close, positive relationships with their fathers and negative feelings toward their mothers, whom they described as cold, rigid, dominating, and critical. Four of these mothers were psychotic periodically and had been in and out of mental hospitals as their daughters grew up. Of the 25, 8 reported feeling closer and more positive toward their mothers and afraid of their fathers. Most of the women reported being attracted to older men who were authority figures. Only a few of the women stated that they tended to choose men weaker than themselves. None felt that she had had an egalitarian relationship with a man and only a few indicated that such a relationship would be desirable. Almost all stated directly that they preferred an authoritarian man. Most preferred male to female friendships and indicated that having sex with their therapists made them feel they were very "special" and it was a validation of their self-worth.

Attitudes of low self-regard characterized the descriptions of their relationships with men, with physical attraction identified as the basis for most of their involvements. Some of the women reported abusive relationships with their sexual partners, and they also had had such relationships with their fathers.

Belote's sample of 25 women appears to consist of middle-risk-type patients. However, it should be pointed out that all of these studies that hypothesize about patients' premorbid personality based on samples of patients who were traumatized may be in error. Descriptions of the process of sexualized therapy by former patients (Freeman and Roy 1976; Plasil 1985; Walker and Young 1986) indicate that the treatment eroded their sense of self and promoted dependency on the therapist. Post-hoc evaluation of the patients' personality as other-directed or as having a dependent personality may therefore be describing a result rather than a cause. Further research is needed in this area.

An alternative to the societally engendered pathology described by Chesler, Belote, and D'Addario are theories of etiology that hypothesize Oedipal or pre-Oedipal origins.

Freud's theory of the etiology of hysterical conversion (1953) stressed Oedipal conflicts and oral fixation. Reich (1951) agreed with this basic tenet of oral needs and underlined the dependence on others for approval and the need for affection and nurturance rather than sex. Marmor (1953) added to the orality the unstable, weak ego, which is very suggestible and can cease symptomatology quickly. Wolowitz (1970) clarifies that these hysterical individuals attempt to find in men the nurturance they missed in their own mothers, and cannot receive from other women due to disappointment they have experienced in the original mothering experience. As mentioned above, the women in the Belote study described their mothers negatively and were emotionally closer to their fathers. Wolowitz explains that in their frantic effort to gain love and attention these individuals sacrifice feelings of realness, lose themselves in the roles that they play, and experience resultant feelings of falseness, emptiness, and loneliness.

It is clear why patients experiencing this emptiness and loneliness might be at risk for involvement with their therapists. They seek power and survival through alliance with a man whom they perceive as strong, powerful, and caring. To achieve that alliance they use weakness, helplessness, and attractiveness to win the love they are lacking and to exercise control over the source of that love. Belote hypothesizes that because such women fear hostility and desire security they deny their own needs and suppress their aggression in favor of pleasing the therapist; however, denying their own needs causes resentment that may be expressed through becoming nonorgasmic, which many of these patients are. Belote buttresses her argument with: (1) Stekel's study of feminine frigidity, which found that often the main contributing factors of such frigidity are hostility and resentment against the husband and lover, and (2) Bardwick's statement that passive aggressive behavior is a culturally normative part of the female sex role. Belote (1974, p. 112) concludes that it is also possible that some women hold back sexually with a man as a way of gaining power over him in a male-dominated world, which allows her few legitimate or acceptable ways of gaining power.

An alternative dynamic explanation for patients' sexual involvement with therapists was provided by L. G. Stone (1980), who hypothesized that severe anxious attachment and weak ego functioning would increase vulnerability to such sexualized relationships with a therapist. In contrast to the theorists mentioned above who emphasize the Oedipal roots of transference and the incestuous nature of the therapist-patient sexual dyad, Stone follows theoretical models pioneered by Greenacre (1954), Spitz (1956), Thompson (1946), and Blum (1973), which propose that such sexual involvement represents a pre-Oedipal need to merge with the mother. These theorists contend that the transference re-creates an early relationship between mother and child and that it promotes repetition of basic attachment experiences. The patient reacts in therapy as she did with the mother (Masterson 1976). The development and direction of the therapy is based on the patient's original separation/individuation experiences. Stone hypothesizes that the patient becomes sexually involved with the therapist in order to preserve the symbiotic attachment, deny feelings of separateness, and defend against object loss. She contends that these women are more vulnerable to sexual involvement with their therapists as a result of a disturbance in separation/individuation that has adversely affected ego functioning and contributed to anxious, clinging attachments to significant others. Stone specifies that the child compromises her needs in order to avoid the mother's punishment for the child's attempt to separate from her. In an effort to defend against feeling separate from the mother, the child clings and attempts to perpetuate a symbiotic attachment. Consequently, clinging is perpetuated and autonomous ego functioning is stifled. During the Oedipal period the child combines her natural desire for physical affection from her father with her unresolved, underlying need for symbiotic union and finds that sex may provide fulfillment of both. Since the patient reacts in therapy as she did with the mother during critical phases of separation/individuation, Stone reasons that these patients attempt to reestablish symbiotic union with their therapists through sexual contact. The sexual fusion enables the woman to deny feelings of separateness from her therapist in much the same way she denied feelings of separateness from the mother during pre-Oedipal development.

Stone's dissertation attempts to obtain empirical evidence for this theory. The study was based on a sample of 46 women who had been in therapy with a male therapist (but had terminated this therapy before participating in the study). The women were divided into four categories: 16 who had been sexually intimate with their therapists; 10 who had been sexually propositioned; 10 whose therapeutic relationship had prematurely terminated; and 10 who had successfully completed therapy.

A highly significant relationship was found between group membership and the strength of anxious attachment to the therapist. Women who had been sexually involved with their therapists had scores indicating stronger anxious attachments (more clinging and acknowledged fear of emotional/physical abandonment by their therapists) than women who had experiences in therapy that had not involved sexual contact. Also, women who were sexually involved with their therapists had the strongest anxious attachments to their therapists, mothers, and boyfriends. On the other hand, women who had successfully completed therapy without sexual involvement with their therapists had the weakest anxious attachments to these specific significant others. Through verbal report it was found that the majority of those women who were sexually involved with their therapists sought another therapist after their sexualized therapy encounter. Stone cautions that the therapist who becomes sexually involved with a patient perpetuates her anxious attachment, colludes with her defense against separation, and precludes her individuation.

THE HIGH-RISK GROUP

Although we have no large-scale empirical evidence as yet concerning the premorbid personalities of the high-risk group, there appears to be a large percentage of these women who, as children, experienced incestuous relationships. This is not surprising. Therapist-patient sex has been compared to incest (Marmor 1972) and it is not unlikely that there is a kind of repetition compulsion that characterizes this type of patient's choice of an older, powerful therapist. The same vulnerability exists in the patient as in the child: the loving, trusting, belief that the parent (or parent-figure) is also loving and caring and would not hurt. There is the same feeling of powerlessness on the part of the child-patient: the fear that one cannot exist without the parent's or the therapist's protection and love.

As a child, the incest survivor has a limited repertoire of adjustment patterns available. These patterns that have served well for survival in childhood become ingrained and fixed. The usual incest victim has been involved in a sexual relationship with a person in authority, either father or someone else, over a period of years and has had to keep the secret. She has learned to take the blame for what happened and has learned to exonerate the adult offender. The paternal role is fulfilled by the therapist with whom she is sexually involved. The therapist is assured of a pliable, often pathetically naive, needy patient who will not tell and who will not blame the therapist but who *will* frequently remain in the therapeutic relationship for years, paying for the damage and feeling guilty for causing the inevitable abuse and neglect by the therapist. Even with substantial understanding and support, such women may find it almost impossible to admit to themselves that victimization has occurred.

The abused child learns to accommodate to a continuing outrageous sexual relationship, outrageous whether or not it is gentle, whether or not it is purported to be loving. The same is true of the relationship with the therapist. Sexualizing the therapy is a betrayal of a trusting relationship that requires an altruism, an unselfish involvement that the parent or therapist must have with a child or client in a subordinate or needy position to leave them whole. Temporarily, the incest survivor or the patient tends to disassociate and find ways of redefining what is going on, so that it does not seem so bad. This denial goes on for a period of time and sex becomes almost commonplace. The need to redeem the relationship, to invent something of quality in the relationship, becomes compelling. The search for a nonsexual relationship with a father figure becomes for many survivors of incest an odyssey, a desperate need. The therapist, especially the male therapist, occupies that transference object position of being the potential good father over the potentially incestous father before a word is spoken. Thus, if that therapist betrays this patient it is a double betrayal, and the patient frequently cannot trust again.

Another quality of the incest survivor makes recurrent victimization likely: the quality of fixation at a childlike level, or a regression to a childlike state under stress. Many women who have achieved a relatively stable adjustment under normal circumstances regress under a stressful situation and find that they cannot say no, particularly to someone in authority who is more powerful than they are. Some who have survived an incest experience and who have found the courage to go into therapy are told by their therapists that their problem is that they can't trust men, and must learn to trust by beginning with the therapist. At this point the incest survivor has her clothes off and finds herself in a familiar situation, wondering what there is wrong with her that she is so stupid that she continues to be victimized and so bad since she must be the one who is inviting these things to happen.

Those patients in this high-risk category frequently possess characteristics associated with Histrionic Personality Disorder or Borderline Personality Disorder as set forth in the American Psychiatric Association's *Diagnostic and Statistical Manual* (third edition, 1980) (*DSM-III*). Both syndromes involve substantial disruptions of interpersonal relationships. The theory and research, taken as a whole, indicate that such disorders are the result of long-term developmental processes. Such personality styles may leave these individuals exceptionally vulnerable to exploitation by unprincipled therapists. When such vicitimization occurs, such patients may require repeated hospitalizations or extreme measures to maintain a sufficiently safe environment (for example, helping them to resist suicidal impulses) in the absence of hospitalization.

From clinical experience we have noted that there appears to be an inordinately large number of patients in the high-risk group who report incestuous experiences and subsequent multiple victimization. Research is needed to confirm this hypothesis. The diagnosing and pathologizing of patients who become sexually involved with their therapists is a sensitive issue. There is a danger of blaming the victim by emphasizing preexisting conditions. How much of the damage is iatrogenic and how much is preexisting is difficult to ascertain.

Three fictional examples are cited here that might be considered typical of the high-risk category.

Example 1. A staff psychotherapist on weekend duty at an inpatient psychiatric hospital received a phone call from a woman in a phone booth who said she was referred to him by a former patient. She had just arrived in town, was without funds, had her eight-year-old son with her, and they had had no food the entire day. Could he come out and pick them up and help them find a place to live? The therapist complied, took the mother and child to a neighbor's home to stay over night and lent the woman an extra car. This began a series of demands by the patient that culminated in a sexual relationship. When the therapist responded the woman ran out into the street, tried to throw herself under a car, and was hospitalized as suicidal. Stabilized, she was released, came to see the therapist, and the incident was repeated. This time she killed herself.

Example 2. A hospitalized woman complained to a patients' rights worker that her psychotherapist was overmedicating her with barbiturates and antipsychotic drugs. Investigation revealed that the patient was not psychotic, nor had she ever been so diagnosed, but had been kept on drugs and in the hospital to sexually service the therapist regularly after he made rounds. When she was released she was barely functional.

Example 3. A 45-year-old woman revealed to her therapist that she had been involved with a previous therapist for 20 years. During that time she had performed fellatio on him weekly but they had never had intercourse. She had never had any other sexual contact. Deeply depressed and suicidal, she realized that she had lived a lifetime in sexual servitude.

How do high-risk patients become involved in such miasmas? Many times very disturbed patients do not see themselves as able to cope with life without an umbilical attachment to the therapist. As dreary as life is, they envision catastrophe without the "helping" professional. The more fragile the patient's ego structure, the more vulnerable she or he is. Dependent, delusional, and sometimes even psychotic, these patients have few defenses. Many sexualizing therapists choose such clients for sexual relationships because they evaluate the client as unlikely to disclose information about therapists' unethical behavior. These therapists may prefer confused, vulnerable women who have had a history of being battered or who are deeply depressed and/or psychotic (Bouhoutsos 1984). Such high-risk patients with severe psychological problems suffer more damage than those initially less incapacitated (Feldman-Summers and Jones 1984). Many of these patients do not realize until years later the impact that the sexual involvement with their therapist has had on them. When such awareness occurs it can be overwhelming, especially if the present treating therapist is not knowledgeable about therapist-patient sexual involvement and places the responsibility on the patient (see Chapter 8). Still further traumatization can occur if the patient consults an attorney who concludes that the statute of limitations has been run and the patient is denied restitution and/or requital (see Chapter 10). Multiple victimization of high-risk patients is an unfortunate but not infrequent occurrence.

The schemata presented here dividing patients into low, medium, and high risk should not be considered the last word on the vulnerability of patients. Our theories must be viewed only as promising hypotheses rather than conclusive categorization. Further, even if at some time we are able to construct categories of risk that are both generalizable and validated (by more than one systematic study), there will still be a substantial number of individuals who will not fit the norms.

Having examined some of the factors leading therapists to involve patients in sexual relationships and factors that make patients vulnerable to exploitation by therapists, we now turn our attention to the consequences of therapist-patient sexual intimacy.

5

Consequences of Therapist-Patient Sexual Intimacy

RESEARCH FINDINGS

Although systematically gathered, empirically based data regarding the effects of therapist-patient sexual intimacy have only recently become available, such relationships have traditionally been assumed to be harmful to patients (Boas 1966; Marmor 1972b). Thus, as has been reviewed in Chapter 2, such intimacy has been prohibited by such various sources as the Hippocratic Oath, Freud, the regulations of state licensing boards, and the formal ethical codes of all major mental health disciplines.

A few authors have claimed beneficial results; the majority have found therapist-patient sexual involvement harmful, as shown in Table 3.

McCartney (1966), the best-known protagonist for sexual relationship with patients, sought justification for his position from earlier authors. He quoted Boss's reasoning that

> "the female analysand begins to love the male analyst as soon as she becomes aware that she has found someone for the first time in her life who really understands her and who accepts her even though she is neurotic. She loves him all the more because the analyst permits her to fully unfold her real emotions within the safe relationship of the transference." In none of his writing does Boss put a limit on the extent to which the analysand should be allowed to go on expressing her needs. . . . I have found that 10 to 30 percent require some overt expression. . . . These patients not only want to think or talk about their relationship to the analyst, but also want to experience the newly discovered possibilities in the language of their emotions, as expressed by the body . . . (pp. 228–29).

McCartney referred only to heterosexual involvements. His contention was

TABLE 3. Studies of Beneficial and Harmful Therapist-Patient Sexual Involvement

Author	Date	Number of Cases	
		Beneficial	
McCartney	1966	1,500	
Shepard	1971	11	
		Harmful	
Chesler	1972	11	
Butler	1975	25	
Freeman and Roy	1976	1	
D'Addario	1977	4	
Stone	1980	46	
Burgess	1981	16	
Bouhoutsos et al.	1983	559	
Feldman-Summers and Jones	1984	30	
Vinson	1984	28	
Plasil	1985	1	
		Mixed	
Taylor and Wagner	1976	34	(7 positive, 11 mixed, 16 negative)

that homosexuality was "immature, neurotic and adolescent. If the analysand is a male and the analyst also male, then the patient's treatment should be shifted to a female analyst when overt expression shows itself" (p. 236).

Yet McCartney did not favor marriage between patients and their sexually involved therapists. He mentioned with disdain an instance where a "contemporary analyst" in 1942 was living with his fifth wife, became emotionally involved with his analysand, divorced his wife, and married the patient. There is no mention in his work of the predecessors Reich, Bernfeld, Rado, and Fenichel who married their patients (Chesler 1972, p. 139). McCartney's contention was that "the analyst must mature into the freedom of selfless concern for his patient. . . . It also includes a free relationship of the analyst toward his own sexuality and his own egotism. . . . The patient may improve in an amazingly short time with an emancipated therapist" (pp. 235–236).

McCartney claimed to have conducted over 1,500 psychoanalyses during his 40 years in practice, with 75 percent of his patients having made "good adjustments." Of his adult female analysands, 30 percent expressed some form of Overt Transference, such as sitting on his lap, holding his hand, hugging or kissing him. About 10 percent found it necessary to act-out extremely, such as mutual undressing, genital manipulation, or coitus.

It is not clear if McCartney means that he was sexually involved with 10 percent of the total 1,500 or 10 percent of the 30 percent (45). Nor is it clear whether the 75 percent who improved included the 30 percent who expressed need for Overt Transference. McCartney does not provide specific data regarding the hours devoted to each of the 1,500 cases. However, some rough calculations yield interesting findings.

McCartney refers specifically to 1,500 *psychoanalyses*. Generally, a complete psychoanalysis lasts approximately five years; however, the following calculation uses four years to provide a conservative estimate. Similarly, although the modal number of sessions per week is five, again, four per week will be used to give McCartney the benefit of the doubt. Assuming 48 treatment weeks per year (allowing two weeks for the analyst's vacation and two for the analysand's), four sessions per week for each analysand and assuming four years for each analysis, each of the 1,500 analyses took 768 hours. At 768 hours per analysis, the 1,500 analyses took 1,152,000 hours. Since McCartney claimed that these analyses were conducted over a 40-year period, he apparently spent 28,800 hours per year or (again using 48 weeks per year) *600 hours per week* on these psychoanalyses. McCartney calls the reader's attention to the fact that the analyses constituted only 26 percent of his overall patient load (p. 236)!

Marmor (1972) rejected McCartney's theory, called attention to his poor psychoanalytic training on which this theory was based and pointed out that McCartney was expelled from the American Psychiatric Association.

Unfortunately, empirical research either to prove or disprove benefit or harm has been very difficult to undertake because of the inaccessibility of both therapist and patient populations. Small-scale studies on self-selected individuals responding to newspaper advertisements or "grapevine" requests for subjects have provided most of the information.

An effort to obtain data was made by Taylor and Wagner (1976) who reviewed the literature for every case of therapist-patient sexual involvement, which they then rated for positive, negative, or mixed outcome. They found that 47 percent of the cases were described as having had negative outcomes and 21 percent of their 34 cases were said to have resulted in positive effects. They did not state, however, how many of the cases were based on therapists' reports, which would obviously make these results suspect since they were evaluating their own "methodology." Patients' self-reports can be assumed to have more veracity since they chronicled their own pain and suffering (Freeman and Roy 1976; Plasil 1985; Walker and Young 1986). Vivid descriptions attest the damaging consequences of therapist-patient sexual involvement for these particular patients. The dynamics of the therapist-patient relationships as described are very familiar to therapists who have worked with such patients.

Shepard (1971) interviewed 11 patients who had had sexual relations with their therapists. He indicated that 8 of the 11 reported emotional growth and that the major therapeutic benefit was reassurance of the patient about her desirability (see Chapter 2 for a discussion of Shepard's book). The California study (Bouhoutsos et al. 1983) indicated that this type of reassurance could be initially positive but in most instances this benefit was drastically reversed by the sometimes delayed negative sequelae of the sexual therapist.

Other studies on small numbers of subjects have attempted to assess both positive and negative outcomes of therapist-patient sexual involvements. D'Addario (1977; see also Durre 1980) found that the sexual involvement was "detrimental, if not devastating" to patients. The sexualized relationships were not satisfying to four women in the study and their original dysfunctions were not cured. Sexual dysfunction was also present in the therapists. Terminations of the relationships were traumatic to the women. There were feelings of rage, hurt, loneliness, and abandonment. All four of the women sought new therapists to recover from the trauma as well as for assistance with the original problem, but they also displayed a surprising amount of denial, rationalization, and understanding of the therapists' problems.

Butler (1975) reported that 95 percent of the 25 therapists she studied who were sexually involved with their patients reported feelings of fear and guilt. Only 40 percent sought help, usually from a friend or colleague.

Chesler's (1972) subjects reported they felt "abandoned" and "mistreated" by their therapists with whom they were sexually involved. Two of the women were severely depressed, one attempted suicide, and the husband of one woman committed suicide after learning of the sexual contact.

Burgess (1981) interviewed women who were involved with their gynecologists and her findings were very similar to those described by researchers of psychotherapist-patient sex. All of the 16 women reported feeling "dirty, humiliated, degraded, embarrassed and nauseated" by the sexual contact. Feelings of anger were reported by 25 percent of the women, and many blamed themselves for the occurrence, developing an aversion to gynecological health care as a result (p. 1338).

Feldman-Summers and Jones (1984) studied 30 women divided into three groups, 20 of whom had had sex with their therapists, 10 as a comparison group, who had not. Of the 20 who had, 19 reported that the impacts were entirely negative. There were three major findings: (1) women who have had sexual contact with their therapists report more anger and mistrust of men and therapists and more psychosomatic symptoms one month after therapy than do comparable women who have not had sexual contact with their therapists; (2) the impacts of sexual contact with one's therapist are not significantly different from the impacts of sexual contact with other health care practitioners (that is, physicians); and (3) severity of the impact of the sexual relationship can be predicted by prior vulnerability and by the martial status of the practitioner. That is, patients who already have severe problems will suffer more damage from a sexual relationship with a therapist than those who are not as vulnerable to begin with. Sexual contact with a married therapist apparently produces additional stress—perhaps guilt and anxiety—which may aggravate the preexisting condition of the patients. Thus if the client is troubled to begin with and the therapist is married, substantially more damage will accrue.

The first large-scale study on the consequence of patient-therapist sexual involvement was done in 1983 (Bouhoutsos et al.). Information was requested from all licensed psychologists in California (N = 4,385 in 1978) about patients reporting sexual involvement with a previous therapist. The study examined the effects on patients and on the therapy process. Although the return rate was low (16 percent), the study was valuable in that it provided large amounts of data. Limited by a truncated sample (those patients not returning to therapy were not included), information was nonetheless available on 559 patients. Of these, 90 percent were described by their subsequent therapists to have suffered negative consequences of some type from their sexual involvement with their previous therapists.

Personality was reported to have been adversely affected in one-third of the cases; for example, patients became more despondent, less motivated, their social adjustment was impaired, or they became significantly more emotionally disturbed. In some instances drug or alcohol use increased; 11 percent of the 559 patients were hospitalized. There were even instances of suicide (1 percent of the cases reported).

Among the one-fourth of the cases for whom sexual, marital, or intimate relationships worsened, mistrust of the opposite sex increased, the marriage and/or family were negatively affected, and sexual relationships were often impaired. Half of the 559 cases reported had problems in recommencing therapy: patients were suspicious and mistrustful of therapists, had difficulty establishing a new relationship, were extremely cautious in choosing a new therapist, or did not return to therapy "for a long time." However, a few sought therapy from another therapist right away to resolve the conflict that had been engendered. Just as in the Feldman-Summers and Jones study, some patients remained emotionally committed to the previous therapist. Some wanted a clear commitment of "no sex" before entering therapy again, and some were afraid that their new therapist would not believe what had happened to them. The more intense the sexual involvement, the greater the likelihood that patients had difficulty returning to therapy rather than quickly seeking help. A high percentage of those who progressed only as far as talking about having sexual relations immediately sought help from another therapist.

Who initiated the sexual relationship was related to adverse effects on the patient's emotional, social, and sexual adjustment and to the therapy. When the therapist initiated sexual intimacies, the patient was more adversely affected and the previous therapy ended or suffered interference in almost all of the cases. When the patient initiated sexual intimacies the patient was adversely affected in only a little over one-third of the cases and the previous therapy ended or suffered interference in three-fourths of the cases. Positive effects, although rare, were more likely to be found when the patient alone or the patient and therapist mutually initiated sexual relations; however, it should be noted that these positive effects subsequently turned to negative effects in many instances.

"When sexual intercourse begins, therapy ends," concludes the Bouhoutsos California study (p. 194). Once sexual activity began, therapy ended immediately for one-third of the patients; further, for one-third of the cases, the onset of sexual intimacies was within the first few sessions, and for three-fourths it occurred within the first year. "Hence a sizable number of patients did not have the benefits of psychotherapy for their original problems, and added to those problems were the complications of a sexual relationship" (p. 194). Control of the course of therapy appeared to pass out of the hands of the therapist once sexual intimacy occurred. At the very least, the therapist appeared to be limited in his or her ability to help the patient.

An interesting dimension was added by a recent study (Vinson 1984) which, while small (N = 28), included male patients (N = 6). Participants were given a 20-item symptom checklist and asked to identify symptoms they experienced before therapy, during the period of greatest stress after termination, and at present. The symptoms that most troubled all of the subjects at the period of greatest stress were depression, alienation from friends and family, hopelessness, and emotional numbness. The female subjects experienced nine times greater increase in symptoms than the male subjects. By the time of the interview the female subjects had returned to their earlier baseline level. The male subjects had 13 times fewer symptoms at the time of the interview than they did at a characteristic pretherapy period. Over half of the women experienced severe disruption of interpersonal relationships, continuing feelings of guilt, shame, and hopelessness, and disruption of cognitive functioning (for example, memory lapses, trouble concentrating, and perseverating thoughts). The male subjects did not perceive their lives as disrupted as did the female subjects during the two-year period following the end of the sexualized therapy. Two-thirds of the female subjects reported sexual difficulties, marked withdrawal from friends, major weight gain and loss, and less social activities or recreational pursuits, thus indicating a severe disruption of their lives.

A high 79 percent of the subjects (in contrast to 90 percent reported by Stone 1980) sought further therapy after the end of the sexualized therapy.

For about three-fourths of these, the primary issue for that therapy was the previous therapy, but several could not bring themselves to tell the subsequent therapists about their sexual involvement even though they recognized that their return to therapy was primarily because of the damage they had suffered. In all, 86 percent of the subjects in the study found the subsequent therapy affected by the sexual relationship with the previous psychotherapist.

Most (86 percent) of the female subjects evaluated the sexualized therapy as very negative. In those instances where there were positive evaluations, the gains were made before the sexual contact (Vinson 1984, p. 116). In contrast, male and homosexual subjects described their experiences as positive. The most commonly mentioned impact of the therapy was that the original problems for which they sought therapy were either ignored or made worse, and that they became sexually inhibited or blocked. Four female subjects indicated that their serious suicide attempts and subsequent hospitalization were the direct outcome of their confusion, panic, guilt, and anger engendered by the sexual relationship with the psychotherapists. Three subjects called it "rape," two called it a "kind of incest." In explanation, each of the five women mentioned both the power imbalance and the violation of trust they had experienced.

Overall, the balance of the empirical findings is heavily weighted in the direction of serious harm resulting to almost all patients sexually involved with their therapists. From patients' own assessments as well as those of subsequent therapists, a substantial patient population sustains damage from sexual involvements with therapists.

CLINICAL FINDINGS

Many of the patients who become involved sexually with their therapists and who subsequently undertake legal remedies are labeled borderline and some are identified as suffering from Post-Traumatic Stress Disorder (PTSD). In fact, 64 percent of her sample were identified by Vinson (1984) as suffering from PTSD as defined by *DSM III* (American Psychiatric Association 1980).

Frequently this diagnosis is made by the subsequent therapist after such patients reenter therapy, or when court-appointed psychologists are asked to evaluate the patient in the context of a suit against the previous therapist. Other requests for patient evaluation may be made to establish the individual's suitability to participate in a support group. A characteristic each of these evaluations has in common is the inordinate distress of the patient and the resistance to testing. This resistance to testing is frequently based on mistrust, and this suspicion is completely understandable. These people have been betrayed on the deepest level, and their refusal to go along with the suggestions of yet another professional makes sense in light of their history. In fact, this assertive questioning—of which they may have been incapable in their previous relationships with therapists—may be a sign of health.

The Minnesota Multiphase Personality Inventory (MMPI) profiles may show extreme distress and dysfunction. It is not unusual to see signs that would contraindicate admission into group treatment (see Chapter 6). In such cases, a valid interpretation of the results of the MMPI and other psychological tests such as the Rorschach, Thematic Apperception Test (TAT), and Millon Clinical Multiaxial Inventory (MCMI), can be made only in light of the individual's history by a psychologist trained and experienced in diagnosis and treatment and for whom the assessment of patients who have been sexually intimate with a previous therapist is an area of authentic expertise.

In addition to diagnostic problems, several clinical issues have emerged from descriptions by subsequent therapists (Sonne et al. 1985; Schoener, Milgrom, and Gonsiorek 1983). For many patients there may be no data deriving from formal testing and assessments performed prior to the sexual involvement with the therapist. Without such baseline data, the assessment of the damage that was due to the sexual involvement becomes more complex and difficult.

The usual clinical picture includes a loss of trust, poor self-concept, problems with expression of anger, loss of confidence in the the patient's own judgment, feelings of guilt, ambivalence about the damaging relationship, and difficulty in establishing a relationship in any subsequent therapy.

It may be that the sequelae of therapist-patient sexual involvement form a distinct clinical syndrome for the patient, with both acute and chronic phases. Aspects of the Therapist-Patient Sex Syndrome (Pope 1985a; 1986b) include: (1) ambivalence, (2) guilt, (3) feelings of isolation, (4) feelings of emptiness, (5) cognitive dysfunction (especially in the areas of attention and concentration, frequently involving flashbacks, nightmares, intrusive thoughts, and unbidden images), (6) identity and boundary disturbance, (7) inability to trust (often focused on conflicts about dependence, control, and power), (8) sexual confusion, (9) lability of mood (frequently involving severe depression), (10) suppressed rage, and (11) increased suicidal risk. The syndrome bears similarities to aspects of borderline (and histrionic) personality disorder, posttraumatic stress disorder, rape response syndrome, reaction to incest, and reaction to child or spouse battering. The appearance of some of these symptoms may be substantially delayed.

Two continuing programs are providing information about these clinical findings: the Walk-In Counseling Center of Minneapolis and the

Post-Therapy Support Group (PTSG) of the University of California, Los Angeles. (See Chapter 6, for a more detailed description of these two programs.) Perhaps the most universal symptom has been the *loss of trust* in therapists, in the legal and professional ethics systems, in the licensing functions, and in the training institutions in which the therapists were educated. Most patients have experienced not only the original trauma with the therapist but continuing upset because of the unresponsive bureaucracies, the delays, the flawed adjudication processes, the constant retelling of the story, the questioning attitudes of the attorneys, the probing into their lives, and the general feeling that *they* are the ones "on trial" rather than the therapists who abused them.

Many of the patients have doubts about the sincerity of the staff of the projects, especially if research is being done. They voice suspicion that they are being used as "guinea pigs" or that the therapists are once again getting *their* needs met. Other accusations were the the the therapists in the PTSG were students and "might be getting credit" for the course or that they were "practicing" on the group members and were not "real" therapists. (The therapists, all advanced graduate students or licensed psychologists, are unpaid and do not receive course credit.) Many resented having to take the MMPI, which they viewed as a screening device, and some group members asked the leaders if they were also willing to take it (Sonne et al. 1985). (All therapists acknowledged having taken it many times.)

Other areas of discomfort were confidentiality, emotional display, touching, and meeting outside the group. Scrupulous attention was given to maintain clear, consistent, and open communications with group members, with very firm boundaries.

Perhaps the most sensitive area was the feeling on the part of group members that since they believed that they had shown poor judgment in choosing the therapist with whom they became sexually involved and who had subsequently betrayed them, they could not trust their own feelings or judgments again. This was a constant source of concern. There was repeated questioning of their own motives and a tendency either (1) to abandon responsibility for themselves and their children completely, turn everything over to someone in authority whom they could not trust, and feel resultantly anxious; or (2) to refuse any kind of help and intervention where it was necessary, and suffer resultant depression and helplessness. Either was destructive and painful.

Many of these patients suffer from PTSD. Many who are seriously traumatized have literally spent lifetimes undoing the damage it has caused. In many instances the trauma becomes the focal point of their existence and they live and relive the scenes of seduction and involvement. In contrast to individuals who have experienced PTSD over war injuries, victims of sexual intimacy with therapists are afraid to reveal their feelings of guilt and betrayal and cannot talk with relatives and friends and in this way find support. They cannot share their views of themselves as stupid and/or seductive. Those who have finally ventured to talk with family and friends, or even with subsequent therapists, frequently find that they are blamed for what occurred, so there is a constant cycle of retraumatization. Consequently, patients withdraw from friends and family because their depression or upset is poorly tolerated when its cause is not understood. Frequently such patients have sleep disturbances, and when they are awake they are obsessed by their self-questioning and self-blame.

Often their lives center around the incident and everything else is subordinated. Marriages fail and children are neglected in the wake of the trauma. The patients become preoccupied, introspective, and mistrustful. Sometimes they are blocked from seeking further therapy, since they tend to generalize and hold all therapists to blame for what occurred. The changes in personality frequently provoke anxious, concerned, or angry responses from those in the immediate family. Frequently there is a change in life-style when they are unable to work and there are resultant monetary problems. There are frequent sexual problems with spouses, with the victim losing desire for closeness and sometimes even a repugnance for sexual contact with the spouse. Fear and frustration alternate with anger and irritability. Fears are frequent; for example, the fear that the therapist with whom they were involved will kill them to avoid a lawsuit. The need for constant reassurance strains the tolerance of family members and ostracizes the victim from even minimal support. Clinically, patients may complain of tension, apprehension, dissociation, fatigue, lassitude, lack of motivation, depression, and/or anxiety. There may be frequent tears or numbness and an inability to cry. Despair and pessimism may be so powerful that functioning is severely limited. The deterioration of familial relationships, inability to work, self-blame, and self-hate may continue and worsen with time unless there is intervention; if there is no intervention, these are the patients at risk for suicide.

EFFECTS OF THERAPIST-PATIENT SEXUAL INVOLVEMENT ON THE THERAPIST

Just as patients have lost their spouses and children as a result of involvement with their therapists, so have therapists in turn had their families leave them. Following are some examples that, while fictitious, represent common situations.

Example 1: A two-career mental health professional couple. The husband-therapist left his wife-therapist of three decades to pursue an affair with a patient who had come with her husband for marital counseling. So two families, with a total of five children, were disrupted and thrown into chaos. The wife of the therapist recognized the disaster for what it was: mid-life crisis on the part of her husband and boredom for the housewife patient. Powerless to change the husband's obsession with the patient, the woman therapist sought a divorce. The therapist married his patient. After a two-year "honeymoon" and the loss of his practice and his family, the therapist attempted suicide.

Example 2: In an instance of therapist-patient sexual involvement that led to a lawsuit, the therapist claimed the patient seduced him. He said that he had wanted to do something nice for that patient, to make him feel better about himself and about life. Instead of being grateful for the caring and the nice remarks, the patient was increasingly demanding and negativistic. He also did not pay his bills. The therapist said that he had become angry about the lack of appreciation and the failure to pay and had turned over the account to a collection agency. In reality, the therapist wanted to be cared for as much as the patient. When the patient did not do so, the therapist abused the patient by refusing to see him. By turning over the bill to the agency and dunning the patient, the therapist's anger provoked the patient to complain and the therapist was brought to trial.

Example 3: The therapist needed power and hypnotized her patient into acquiescing to the therapist's plan for her. She kept the patient in bondage for 20 years by giving her drugs so that she would provide the therapist with sexual weekly favors. The therapist made the pact with the patient by threatening that if she revealed the arrangement she would lose the relationship and the patient was so addicted that she couldn't tell anyone. The therapist was vindictive, hostile, and wanted to hurt the patient. She saw the patient as subhuman and denigrated her, telling her that she could never function alone and that she was totally undesirable. Relief came only when the arrangement was exposed. The patient's spouse became aware and instituted divorce action. The patient told another staff physician who pointed out that the situation was harmful. The patient sued the therapist.

Example 4: The therapist was an alcoholic. He encouraged a male patient to sleep with the therapist's wife to relieve some of the patient's concerns about his own sexual identity. Therapy became unworkable because of the jealousy and role confusion.

Example 5: The therapist was vulnerable and had a very poor self-image. Her husband had left her and her patient was very attractive and seductive. She halted the therapy but continued to see the patient after hours and in his apartment. He owed her a great deal of money at the time the sexual relationship started and after the relationship cooled she turned the bill over to a collection agency. He filed an ethics action and a civil suit.

Example 6: An assistant working with a therapist to accumulate hours necessary for licensure began to feel attracted to a woman in her practice.

She felt uncomfortable about taking it up with her supervisor and did not mention to him what was occurring. Gradually she became sexually involved with the patient. When the relationship ended the patient filed a complaint with the licensing board against the assistant. Not only was the assistant deprived of her position, the supervisor was suspended, since he was responsible for the work of the assistant.

EFFECTS ON SIGNIFICANT OTHERS

A tragic by-product of therapist-patient sexual involvement is the breakup of families whose members are the "innocent bystanders" of these relationships. Frequently the husband comes to marriage counseling to avoid the breakup of a marriage and is cuckolded by the therapist; either he divorces his wife when he learns of her infidelity, or she divorces him to devote herself to care for the therapist. The children of this couple often stay with the husband—resentful, angry, deprived of many years of normal emotional growth that they can never replace. A variation is a mother-daughter involvement with the same therapist, which results in alienation when either hears about the involvement of the other. Often it is a period of many years before families can deal with feelings of inadequacy and failure engendered by the alienation.

Even after termination of the sexualized therapy relationships the damage frequently cannot be repaired. The denouement takes years, and if lawsuits are filed, the final resolution may require that most of the lifetime of some families be taken up dealing with the therapist-patient relationship and its sequelae. The guilt feelings experienced by the parents may be lifelong as may the effects on either spouse and/or children. Often there are other relatives involved—parents, grandparents, or even aunts and uncles—who are asked for financial support as a result of the collapse of the family structure and who are pulled into the resultant catastrophe. Usually they do not understand the ramifications of what happened and become resentful and angry, and family members are alienated from one another.

Employers, roommates, friends, co-workers, fellow students—the lives of all can be affected by a patient's or therapist's involvement. The ripple effect can touch a family, agency, university department, or business. Therapist-patient sex not only causes private misery; frequently it constitutes public calamity.

6

Modalities of Support, Advocacy, Mediation, and Therapy

AVOIDING ADDITIONAL TRAUMATIZATION

Patients who have been sexually involved with their therapists need special treatment by their subsequent therapists. When a patient tells us about such an occurrence we have the opportunity to intervene in a supportive, therapeutic way if we are sensitive to the issues involved, or we can traumatize our patients yet again and deepen the iatrogenic wounds they have sustained. What might be acceptable or even desirable therapy with other patients can decimate someone who has been through a sexual experience with a former therapist. Following are two fictional examples.

Example 1: Mary had been molested by her brother at age 8. Her mother refused to believe her, but subsequently took her to church, made her kneel for several hours and confess to the priest how evil she was for "leading her brother astray." As an adult Mary sought help from a therapist who told her that she had to work through the trauma of that earlier incident. He proceeded to undress her and have intercourse with her as she stood immobilized and terrorized in front of him. After a few months when Mary was able to tell her family physician what had occurred, he referred her to a psychiatrist colleague. The psychiatrist accused her of being seductive and placed the responsibility on her for the sexual incident. By the time she was seen by the subsequent therapist she was so angry and resentful of all therapists that it was months before any trust could be built up or the anger could be sufficiently dealt with so that therapy could begin. It is likely that treatment in this instance will take many years and it may never be possible to assuage the pain. Placing this type of responsibility on the patient is simply not good therapy. These patients are already guilt-ridden, with deep feelings of inadequacy, shame, and self-doubt. To burden them with additional guilt is antitherapeutic. In the therapeutic relationship, it is always ultimately the therapist's responsibility to ensure that sexual contact with the patient never occurs.

Example 2: Joan told her therapist that she had been sexually involved with a previous therapist, and that she knew he had had sex with other patients. The therapist was visibly shaken and asked Joan for his name. Joan refused to give the name, saying that she did not want to get him in trouble, that he was going through a difficult time since he was getting a divorce and that it would hurt him too much to know that Joan had reported him. The new therapist told Joan she had a responsibility for the other women with whom he was involved and that he should be reported immediately. The feelings of guilt and the ambivalence toward the previous therapist plunged Joan into a deep depression and she was unable to function. She could not file a complaint, and resultantly felt that she could not return to the new therapist.

Advocacy for patients by subsequent therapists who are told by their patients about sexual involvement with a prior therapist is often difficult and sometimes ill advised. As mentioned in Chapter 7, these subsequent therapists may feel angry or punitive toward members of their profession who have taken advantage of patients, as in Example 2. They may push patients to take precipitous action. Subsequent therapists may also feel frustrated about not being able to report the case if their patient does not wish to take any action, especially when they know other patients are being harmed. Nonetheless, confidentiality forbids the disclosure of the unwilling patient even if there are other members of the public at risk. Despite the concern of the subsequent therapist, there is frequently nothing that can be done unless a patient will sign a complaint.

SELF-HELP AND ADVOCACY GROUPS

One of the reasons patients are not willing to file is their feeling that they are unique in having been betrayed or used. When they find that others have had similar experiences they are frequently able to take a step toward lodging a complaint. Most of the peer support groups have advocacy for victims as one of their purposes. Currently there are several self-help groups in various parts of the country founded by ex-patients who have been "victims" of therapists.

Self-help groups are a vital resource in the array of potential services for those who have been sexually exploited by their therapists. First, as anyone who is acquainted with Alcoholics Anonymous, Cocaine Anonymous, Debtors Anonymous, Gamblers Anonymous, and similar twelve-step programs knows, self-help groups can provide an empathetic, nurturing, and "knowing" environment of others who have "been there." Each patient or ex-patient who describes intensely personal accounts of sexual intimacies with a therapist knows that each listener can personally relate in some way to the experience. Each listener has lived through a similar horror. Each is engaged in a similar struggle to "pick up the pieces," perhaps even just to go on living. This network of people who have suffered a similar catastrophic event can help overcome the sense of isolation and the impulse to withdraw.

Second, self-help groups offer the opportunity for *appropriate* friendships among those involved. Participants can meet for lunches and dinners, accompany each other to parties and other social events, and engage in other activities which would be unethical and clinically destructive were they to involve a therapist and patient.

Third, twelve-step programs are free. A preamble read aloud at the opening of every meeting states clearly that there are no dues or membership fees. Those who paid fees to a therapist and were abused by that therapist may be reluctant to pay money to yet another professional.

Fourth, survivors of therapist-patient sex who are too terrified even to be in the room with a mental health professional are able to obtain help from non-professionals. Trust may never be easy, but some may only be able to talk about their pain and to reach out for help among a group which specifically excludes professionals (at least professionals in the role of professionals; some therapists may themselves be sexually abused by their therapists and need, for a variety of reasons, a self-help group).

Mistrust of persons of the offending gender and anger against therapists in general often motivate the patient to seek a self-help group rather than psychotherapy in the hope of finding support and safety with other "victims." Frequently such patients entering a group very clearly state that they do not wish to have psychotherapy, that they want only support.

Any anger at therapy or therapists is understandable for most of the members have been severely damaged by therapists. While the groups were founded primarily for support, most also are involved in advocacy functions such as supporting legislation or informing the public about the exploitation of patients by the therapeutic disciplines. It is not unusual for members to reject any assistance summarily from therapists who express concern and a willingness to help. Often those therapists are met with distrust, but frequently that distrust is accompanied by a request for assistance, and indication of the ambivalence that characterizes the self-help group members' feelings for their former therapists. It is important for professionals working with these expatients to be sensitive to their own countertransference and to be able to deal with it. Professionals frequently become angry and respond negatively to these patient groups which makes it difficult for professionals and self-help groups to work together on common goals.

The Walk-In Counseling Center in Minneapolis appears to have successfully bridged the gap. It provides advocacy as well as counseling. Begun in 1974, the clinic has provided individual and group counseling as well as assistance in filing complaints against therapists. Over the ten years approximately 300 patients have been seen, and about half of those have filed complaints with either ethics committees, administrative agencies that have a licensing function, or civil courts.

Another group that provides assistance to patients is the Patients' Rights Advocates organization, which has as its primary function the protection of patients hospitalized in state institutions. In some areas, Advocates are also willing to assist private patients in dealing with victimization by a therapist. For patients like one found by Medicaid investigators in a Western hospital who was kept on drugs and institutionalized to provide sexual favors for her therapist, having such information could have been crucial. For example, in California in 1983 handbooks passed out to all patients in institutions were amended to state unequivocally that patients have the right not to be sexually abused by other patients, by staff, or by the therapists of the institution. Although this appears to be a simple statement, it is important to enunciate this principle for staff as well as patients. Too often staff members are aware of such exploitation but are hesitant to do anything about reporting it. In Minnesota such reporting is now mandatory. In 1980 Minnesota enacted the Vulnerable Adults Act, which established the illegality of any mistreatment of patients (including sexual involvement) who were defined as "vulnerable." This controversial legislation mandated reporting of such illegal activity over the objection of the patient. Legislation subsequently clarified that this law did not obtain for outpatient care. Many objections have been raised to mandatory reporting.

Of primary concern is the breach of confidentiality that is necessitated by compulsory reporting. In most states mental health professionals are already required to report child and elder abuse as well as serious threats of violence. In particular this patient population that has already lost trust in the professions would thus be subject to still another betrayal of the confidentiality privilege. Still another objection to the Vulnerable Adults Act was raised by some women's groups who were reluctant to define patients as vulnerable; since most of the patients sexually involved with their therapists are women (Bouhoutsos et al. 1983), this supports a stereotype of women as helpless, dependent, and vulnerable. An opposing argument is that without mandatory reporting by the mental health professionals who are told by their patients of their involvement with a prior therapist, the current situation will continue; 4 percent of the patients who are damaged report and of those, 2 percent complete their cases (Bouhoutsos et al. 1983). Thus it is obvious to therapists who are contemplating becoming sexually involved with their patients that they are very unlikely to be apprehended.

Strong positive arguments have been advanced for mandatory reporting (George 1985, p.454): "The fundamental right of privacy inherent in every individual sometimes must yield to a compelling state interest." George emphasizes that professional organizations have not controlled psychotherapist-patient sex and that legal deterrents are ineffective. He calls for a statute requiring reporting by the subsequent therapist, which would result in the suspension or revocation of licenses and/or criminal prosecution by local district attorneys. Thus the "risk of harm to unsuspecting citizens who many require mental health services in the future would be reduced" (p. 454). George is careful to point out that these future patients are not at risk because they are mentally infirm or per se vulnerable, but "their vulnerability stems from the uniqueness of the psychotherapy relationship and the childlike, dependent position that they assume upon subjecting themselves to mental health treatment" (p. 456). Despite his enthusiastic support of mandatory reporting, however, George recognizes the dangers inherent in requiring the subsequent therapist to name the patient. Thus the proposed statute permits withholding the names of the parties if "reporting would result in 'unusual injury' to the patient" (p. 456). This controversial proposal is still the subject of heated debate among professionals.

Another area of controversy is the effort to criminalize therapists' sexual involvements with patients. Currently, only Minnesota and Wisconsin have such legislation (See Chapter 11) and some groups in California have been attempting to pass such legislation for the past three years through bills proposed by a former school psychologist, now a state senator. The bill has been consistently defeated. At least one self-help group has been very active in support of the bill and some of its members have indicated that such advocacy has been therapeutic for them in that it has allowed direct expression of anger, not only at the offending therapists but at the system that allows them to continue practice with impunity.

Can one be both advocate and therapist? This sensitive area deserves exploration. It is difficult to remain impartial and unmoved when dealing with a patient who has suffered iatrogenic damage. Yet, if we are angry and punitive we may push too hard and patients who are not ready to take action may feel that they have failed or displeased us (see Chapter 7). It is commonplace for the working through of the trauma to take years of painstaking effort. Frequently the patients are protective of the therapists who damaged them, unwilling to identify them and prone to shoulder—regardless of the facts—the responsibility for the sexual relationship. Many still hope that the relationship can be repaired if only they can learn to be less demanding or more understanding or more giving. For some it seems that it may never be possible to speak openly about what occurred, shamed as they are about their supposed role in what happened. These are the patients who would be unable to undergo an ethics or administrative hearing let alone the rigors of a civil suit. For these patients neither advocacy nor self-help groups are appropriate.

MEDIATION

An alternative model has evolved in which patients may elect to face the therapists with whom they have been sexually involved in mediation sessions. This model, originated by the Walk-In Counseling Center of Minneapolis (Schoener, Milgrom, and Gonsiorek 1983) is now being used in California (Bouhoutsos and Brodsky 1985). Modeled after divorce mediation, the session is requested of the current therapist by the patient. The present therapist assesses the readiness of the patient to undergo this type of confrontation and if such meeting is clinically desirable, calls the previous therapist and details the nature of the proposed meeting. The therapist may choose a ''second'' to be present: a colleague, but not an attorney. The subsequent treating therapist is present to assist the patient. The fifth person is the moderator, who clarifies the roles and runs the session. The meeting is to air feelings on both sides, and to facilitate both parties moving on with their lives. All things said are unofficial, but the material that emerges is not privileged and can be used in legal actions if such should be undertaken. The mediation begins by clarifying the purpose of the meeting and establishing the ground rules. The patient is then invited to tell the story from his or her point of view. The sexually involved therapist then responds with his or her version. Contrary to ethics hearings, experience in this type of session has been that there are relatively few disputations of facts. The mediation session has generally been used to express feelings of anger, hurt, disappointment, contrition, concern, and regret. After all participants have had the opportunity to speak, the moderator clarifies, summarizes, and synthesizes.

Is there the possibility that mediation might deter a patient's filing charges by facilitating the discharge of anger and that the sexually abusive therapist might resultantly be allowed to continue involvements with other patients? Or could mediation be used to get evidence for a legal suit or as a false act of contrition (Bouhoutsos and Brodsky 1985)? All of these things are possible. On the other hand, the benefit of such confrontation is the speed with which such a meeting can take place in contrast to the years of waiting for the courts. There is the possibility that the mediation session may enable the participants to get on with their lives. A successful confrontation of the therapist can assist a patient to resolve and dissolve the relationship that otherwise might necessitate putting his or her life on hold. Also, mediation sometimes assists patients to start legal action that they were previously unable to undertake. Sometimes therapeutic gain can result from such sessions.

GROUP THERAPY

Patients who have been sexually involved with their therapists in most cases seek some kind of help after the damage occurs. They apparently do not change disciplines but frequently change their choice of genders of the therapists they consult (Bouhoutsos et al. 1983). It cannot be emphasized enough that the subsequent therapist must be aware of the therapeutic issues and the special needs of this population. The volatility, hypersensitivity, emotional liability, and fragility of these patients make demands on the emotional resources, the time, and the therapeutic skills of the subsequent therapists. When the modality chosen is group psychotherapy there are additional problems.

The Post-Therapy Support Group at the University of California, Los Angeles (UCLA) was founded in 1982 by the authors. It was decided in the planning state that this would not be an advocacy program. Housed in the Psychology Clinic, the program began with a colloquium given by the authors to a group of advanced graduate psychology students who responded with interest to an invitation to participate in the program. Euphemistically named the Post-Therapy Support Group, emphasis was placed on the supportive nature of the project. Licensed psychologist Janet L. Sonne, who is a member of the UCLA clinical faculty, and five advanced graduate students—Debra Borys, Roberta Falke, Valerie Marshall, Buf Meyer, and Tony Zamudio—began the training and committed themselves to a program that offered no credit or compensation. Subsequently psychologists Laurie Astor-Dubin, Allison Parelman and graduate students Sherry Adrian, Delia Magana, David Miranda, and Judy White joined the project. Months of training and planning ensued. Three-hour weekly meetings were held featuring a number of guests who addressed various aspects of therapist-patient sex and the systems that were involved in dealing with the consequences. A senior special investigator for the Board of Medical Quality Assurance explained the complaint process and the preliminary interviews with the complainant and the respondent. A deputy attorney general detailed the administrative law process, the various licensing boards, their structure and function. An anonymous patient who had been sexually involved with a therapist spoke to the group about the emotional impact and the sequelae of her sexual involvement with her therapist. A former chair of the American Psychological Association Ethics Committee addressed ethical issues and the processing of ethical complaints filed by patients who had had sex with their therapists. The founder of a self-help group addressed the question of self-help versus therapy groups. Several psychology diplomates offered information about group work and therapy with survivors of victimization processes. When approximately six months of initial training were completed, we turned our attention to recruitment. Patients were obtained by distributing brochures describing the purpose of the group to community agencies and local therapists. An article in the Los Angeles *Times* resulted in many inquiries, and several televised interviews about the program resulted. As they responded, potential group members were interviewed by the PTSG graduate students. MMPI's were administered in individual sessions. The results were discussed by the project staff and feedback sessions were held with the patients.

We used our assessment sessions to try to determine which patients were in a position to benefit from outpatient group treatment, and which patients might respond better to other approaches (and for whom group therapy might be contraindicated). We made every effort to ensure that those for whom group therapy was not the treatment of choice had access to more appropriate resources. Among those alternative resources was individual therapy either within the clinic (with sliding-scale fees) or with a therapist who was experienced in this area of practice and who maintained an office geographically convenient to the patient.

A major concern was that those patients who were not included in the group would feel rejected. Indeed, patients frequently expressed the feeling that they were being tested to see if they were "worthy" of admission to the group. This sensitive area is one of which all therapists should be aware.

As the project progressed, however, we found that the criteria for admission to the group did not need to be so strict. Some patients who suffered extreme distress and dysfunction, for whom outpatient group therapy would seem to be contraindicated, managed to work quite well within the group context and to benefit substantially from this modality.

All of the group participants were female until the third group began. A male patient applied to join and there were some concerns on the part of project members about how he would be received and how he, as a lone man, might feel in group. Some of the patients in the group expressed discomfort with the idea of including a man as a member of the group, but through discussion and exploration they determined that he was "also a victim" and decided to include him. Whether it was because of this particular individual or the preparation or the character of the group itself, the experience was a very positive one for all involved. We have not as yet included any male project members as group leaders, although we are seriously considering the possibility. We are now beginning the fourth year of the program and the fourth group. Some of the original staff members are still with us, returning from community agencies or internships to donate time.

The PTSG project staff found that consultation with current therapists of patients who were sexually involved with a previous therapist provided an important service to the community. In two instances the current therapists had had no experience with this type of patient and requested consultation by group members. We welcomed the opportunity to provide written material about current research on therapist-patient sexual involvement and to discuss the special needs of this population.

In one instance a young, inexperienced therapist from the community asked if the patient should be transferred to one of the supervisors and we were able to reassure her that the positive relationship that she now had with the patient was crucial in the recovery. It was important to assist the present therapist in understanding the difficulties of establishing the transference relationship and in recognizing the countertransference that arises in so many of these cases. The patient's mistrust of his or her own feelings and suspicion about the motivation of the new therapist is a double bind that can be frustrating to the treating therapist. Since patients feel that they cannot trust their own judgment (and they cannot since they have tangible evidence that their first choice of therapist ended in disaster for them), they must turn to someone else on whom they can rely. Their families generally have not understood the problem and have either denied its existence or have blamed the patient. Since they do not trust men (usually the therapists were male) and do not trust therapists generally, unremitting testing ensues with anger, reproach, threats, demands, and depression. However, growth is often dramatic and may alternate with partial regression. It is frequently helpful to have a consultant as well as someone with whom to share being "on call" for suicidal threats and need for long telephone conversations for support. Dependence is another double-edged sword. These patients are very needy and reach out constantly, but they are angry with their dependency and blame the therapist for encouraging that dependency. Yet if it is withheld, they cannot function and are in danger of suicide. The agonizing nature of these conflicts is a challenge to the resources of both patient and subsequent therapist (see Chapter 8).

A problem that repeatedly surfaced in the PTSG was the continuing ambivalence toward former therapists. Much as an abused child may have positive feelings for the abusing parent and will defend that parent against attack, these patients were sensitive to any derogatory remarks made about their former therapists.

Almost all experienced problems with boundaries, understandable in light of their previous involvement with therapists who violated therapy boundaries. Group members had difficulties setting appropriate boundaries in their relationships with each other, and with their new therapists. For example, one member feared she might slip into a caretaker role in the group at the expense of getting her own needs met (Sonne et al. 1985). Many called each other, needing to talk and gain support, but fearful lest they might overtax the relationship. Others felt guilty when they limited the phone time they made available to group members on request of spouses and/or children. Several revealed that they continued to have difficulties establishing boundaries, and were currently involved with a new therapist, a professor, or a supervisor. Testing of the boundaries set by the group leaders was also frequent. Invitations to dinner, requests for longer sessions, and endless phone calls had to be evaluated in terms of not only the neediness and suicidality but also the desirability of holding to desirable boundaries. Consultation was also very helpful in this area, where many decisions were complex.

Most important was the extreme vulnerability and fragility of these patients, which they themselves experienced. They recognized their need for help but rejected that help. Sophisticated in the language of therapy because of their long exposure to the process, they recognized the typical therapeutic reponses and challenged the group leaders. Reflecting reponses, comments on process, or any kind of confrontation would evoke flashes of anger. Yet group members recognized the complexities and the contradictions involved and could on occasion even sympathize with the group leaders, but basically they rejected the "therapy" model. They were most comfortable when they themselves were talking and when the therapists only made supportive comments. Frequently they spent hours after the sessions talking in the halls outside the therapy room or in the parking structure.

In and outside of the group they would discuss the problems of how much to trust, recognizing that the previously complete trust had been ill-advised. Recognizing that they have to trust someone, they struggled with the question of how far should they trust and how could they assess trustworthiness. Several times there was a growing awareness that they (group members) were responsible for their own growth, that they should open themselves and talk about their feelings in order to get better. But they also needed to feel that they had a choice in doing so.

The group process appeared to follow these patterns:

1. The beginning sessions dealt mostly with a recounting of the traumatic incident. Group members were eager to share their experiences and there was a great deal of support in evidence when the narrator broke into tears in the telling of the story. Emotionally, most of the group members blamed themselves for what occurred and expressed guilt over their role in the sexual relationship. Self-abasement and denigration of their behavior were quite common.

2. As awareness of common patterns began to develop, there was diminution of self-blame, and a growing recognition that the sexual involvement was the therapist's responsibility.

3. Anger and rage began to surface, although positive feelings toward the therapists were also present and caused many emotional outbursts. Some filed charges at this point. Not all of the group members moved to this stage at the same time and those who felt positive feelings for their therapists were challenged by those who were angry. It was continually necessary to emphasize individual differences and the right to make choices about whether or not to take action.

4. Fear, anxiety, and depression began to surface. Those who had filed against their therapists began to have fantasies about being chased, harassed, and even murdered by the previous therapist (such fantasies are particularly understandable in light of the violent threats made by many sexually exploitive therapists). Some fantasized about killing their therapists and were frightened by their own anger. Some would stalk the therapist, watching the windows of the office or speculating on whether the therapist was sexually involved with the patients observed entering the office. Anxiety arose about the depth of the anger felt and about the possibility that there could be acting out and that they could not control their impulses. There was much self-doubt at this point, the feeling that they would never recover from the trauma.

5. The growth of insight became apparent. There was rejection of the previous therapist, the recognition that the sexual involvement was based on the therapist's own personal problems. However, the loss of trust became more acute and there was emergence of skepticism, humiliation, embarrassment, loss of dignity, continued self-blame for having been so easily duped, and so on, but with an intellectual awareness that these feelings were transitory.

6. There was a tentative emergence of trust. A beginning willingness to trust themselves and their own judgment. A recognition of their own power and of their growing independence. A sense of freedom to choose whether to be further involved in working for legislation in the area of patient-therapist sexual involvement or to say no and move on with life without feeling guilty. Group members were able to ask for help and appreciated when it was given, but it had to be given on their terms. Sensitive to the leaders and to each other, the groups were eventually able to build trust, express positive as well as negative feelings, and to go on with their lives. Consensus of the project members is that this kind of specialized clinical work is very difficult but very satisfying, as is evidenced by the longevity of the project.

In addition to the work with the PTSG group, project members frequently were called on to present in-service training to community agencies and continuing education workshops at the conventions of the various disciplines. Empirical research was contemplated initially, but the special sensitivities of group members to possible exploitation and fear of being used for the therapists' own needs precluded that possibility for the present.

Having completed this brief survey of various treatment modalities, we now examine issues faced by virtually all subsequent treating therapists (Chapter 7) and special treatment issues and techniques relevant to individual therapy (Chapter 8).

7

Overall Structuring, Assessment, and the Initial Phase of Treatment

When patients begin opening up about their sexual involvement with a former therapist, it is almost always a moment of great crisis and opportunity. They are likely experiencing a confusing mix of seemingly contradictory emotions. Memory fragments may erupt into awareness, triggering further flashbacks. Thoughts and feelings that have long been suppressed and repressed may come surging back, threatening to overwhelm.

The subsequent therapist who is privy to this process of opening up is likely aware of a special responsibility to help patients through this confusing and frightening time. The sacred trust that a patient bestows upon a therapist has been violated by the previous therapist. The fear of further betrayal is acute. In the midst of this difficult situation, the subsequent therapist must help the patient—often over a very long course of time—come to grips with three major questions: (1) What exactly happened in the patient's relationship with the previous therapist? (2) What are the effects and what does this mean for the patient's life? (3) What, if anything, does the patient want to do about it?

There is no mechanical set of rules that all subsequent therapists can follow at all times with all patients. Each patient is unique, as is each therapist. However, cetain tasks are vital to the process of assessment and recovery. Tasks related to the following 14 issues seem fundamental to effective work with patients who have been sexually involved with a prior therapist:

1. The Therapist's Ability to Listen Openly
2. The Patient's Need to Move at His or Her Own Pace
3. The Legal Context of the Therapy
4. Records

5. Fee Arrangements
6. Biases, Conflicts, and Counter-transference of the Therapist
7. Trust
8. The Patient's Reconstruction of Events

81

The following sections discuss each of these issues.

LISTEN CAREFULLY TO THE PATIENT

Hearing complaints about a colleague is likely to elicit uncomfortable feelings of shock, anxiety, dismay, or disblief. Such feelings may lead a subsequent therapist to screen out further information. The patient may discern, on the basis of the therapist's questions, comments, facial expressions, or body language, that this topic is taboo. The phenomenon is similar to that of some parents who are reluctant to listen to their children reveal that a kindly uncle has made sexual advances. It is also similar to the dynamics that make some therapists seemingly insensitive to their patients' tacit messages of suicidal intent. Therapists must convey their openness and attentiveness to anything the patient has to say.

DON'T CROWD THE PATIENT

While desperately wanting acceptance and support, patients need to move at their own pace. The material that begins to emerge is frequently terrifying, overwhelming. Patients may begin to feel out of control. Feeling pushed or prodded by the therapist is almost always a negative experience. "Breaking through" defenses can have harmful consequences. If patients begin to feel that it is the therapist who will dictate when and how much material will be dealt with, they may feel that their only option is to flee therapy. They need to feel that it is permissible for them not to talk about the subject when they don't feel up to the experience. The new therapeutic situation needs to be one in which the patient first and foremost feels safe and secure. Respect for the patients' decisions about what they will deal with, and the rhythm that is most comfortable and productive for them, is essential.

REVIEW THE LEGAL CONTEXT ACCURATELY AND SPECIFICALLY

It is not only patients but also professionals who are frequently confused about the variety of strictures and responsibilities regarding the content of therapy. Patients, being citizens, possess certain rights to privacy as delineated in constitutional and tort law. Therapists, as professionals, are bound to maintain ethical standards of appropriate confidentiality. Privilege, a distinct but related concept, refers to the power of patients to prevent the disclosure of information. In almost all cases, the privilege belongs to the patients. This is a fact about which some therapists become confused. The privilege belongs to the patient, not to the therapist. The therapist is legally and ethically required to claim the privilege on behalf of the patient in certain instances.

As if all this were not sufficiently complex, both legislatures and courts have, in some instances, designated therapists to act, in effect, as agents for the government or society at large. In such instances therapists must convey to appropriate third parties information about their patients. For example, therapists who determine that their patients are threatening serious harm to another person may be required by the courts or legislatures to notify (without the consent of the patient) the police and/or the intended victim of the risk (Pope in press). Similarly, most states have mandatory child abuse reporting laws. Thus if a therapist forms an opinion from the available data that a patient is abusing a child, the therapist is required to make a report to the appropriate governmental agency.

It is important to discuss such obligations with patients, to ensure that they fully understand the ground rules of therapy. Many patients who have been sexually intimate with a former therapist may assume that there are mandatory or discretionary reporting laws regarding the intimacy. In most states this is not the case. That is to say, information provided about prior sexual intimacies with a therapist is protected by the customary rule of privacy, confidentiality, and privilege. The exceptions to the protection, which vary from state to state, need to be explicitly clarified. In summary, in most states a subsequent therapist cannot disclose a patient's report of sexual intimacy with a previous therapist to any third party without the freely given and fully informed consent of the patient.

When a patient files a complaint, the privilege is generally waived. Thus in the case of a malpractice suit against the previous therapist, the subsequent therapist can be subpoenaed to testify and will have no legal grounds for withholding information about the patient and the therapy. This fact must be fully understood by both patient and therapist at the beginning of treatment. It should not come as a surprise to the patient once he or she decides to file suit.

KEEP APPROPRIATE RECORDS

Because the patient may decide to file a civil suit, a formal complaint to the licensing board, or a complaint to an Ethics Committee, the therapist's notes may become an important source of evidence and information. Therapists must have a well-thought-out system of keeping records in such cases, and must be aware that these records may be reviewed by third parties, many of whom will have neither training nor experience in the mental health field. In addition, given the publicity attendant to many malpractice trials and licensing board actions, the content of the records may become public record. Both therapist and patient should clearly understand the nature of the records that are being maintained and the possible sources of access to those records.

ESTABLISH CLEAR FEE ARRANGEMENTS

This principle, like many of the others, holds for all therapeutic arrangements, but it is particularly important here. If the therapist enters into an agreement to work on a contingency arrangement, a bias may be introduced. This becomes a major issue if the therapist is then called to testify, as an expert witness, in legal procedings. For more detailed discussion of this issue, see Chapter 11 concerning testifying as an expert witness.

CLARIFY PERSONAL BIASES, CONFLICTS, AND COUNTERTRANSFERENCE

Therapist-patient sexual intimacy is such an emotionally charged subject, subsequent therapists may find themselves harboring assumptions or tendencies that can work against the therapeutic process. Some may feel that patients virtually never have a legitimate complaint. They dismiss such complaints as expressions of the patient's transference or pathology, or they minimize the damaging consequences. Others, upon hearing their patients' complain, may be so outraged that they attempt to pressure them into filing formal complaints immediately. Still others may fear that the airing of such complaints in any public forum is likely to give the profession a "black eye" or to raise malpractice rates even further. Still others may try to quiet the patient down, fearing a long and unpleasant involvement in legal proceedings. It is crucial that subsequent therapists become aware of such biases, conflicts, and countertransference and to take effective steps to see that they do not interfere with the therapy.

RECOGNIZE TRUST AS A CENTRAL ISSUE

In some sense it is an almost miraculous occurrence that patients, having been harmed so deeply by a therapist who involves them in sexual intimacies, can summon the courage and trust to seek out a new therapist to attempt to repair the damage. Sometimes this reaching out is born of desperation; perhaps on the verge of suicide, the patient turns to a new therapist as a last chance to stay alive. Whatever the circumstances, the patient's trust in the new therapist will almost always, on some level, be viewed with suspicion and ambivalence by the patient, in light of his or her previous experience.

Patients will often have some suspicion, easily understandable in light of their previous experience, that this new therapy will also, in some way, involve sexual exploitation. Therapists should discuss this issue openly with their patients, stating that no sexual intimacy will occur. Physical touching may be an issue of concern for many patients. Therapists and their patients should agree on appropriate guidelines regarding nonsexual touching—such as handshakes—that are comfortable for both parties and that are in full accordance with clinical and ethical standards. If a patient desires that the therapist never touch him or her, this should be respected. Patients should have good and explicit reason to expect that therapy will provide a safe and secure environment.

LET THE PATIENT DESCRIBE WHAT HAPPENED

Patients often have difficulty putting their experience into words. Especially in initial sessions, they may speak in cryptic and elliptical phrases. Major aspects of the traumatic experience may still reside outside the patient's awareness. These buried memories will almost certainly become accessible to memory eventually, but for the moment they leave major gaps. It is natural for the therapist to "fill in the blanks," or, more technically, to project onto the patient's vague and ambiguous outline the therapist's own ideas about what "really" happened or what "must have" happened. It is critical that therapists not interfere with patients' efforts to reconstruct the experience to the best of their ability.

At times, patients may have an awareness of certain memories but find it difficult to speak them aloud because of intense feelings of shame, guilt, or embarassment. Therapists need to be alert to their patients' reactions to the process of reconstructing the events.

ASSESS AND MANAGE SUICIDAL RISK

Patients who have been sexually intimate with their previous therapists are often in great distress and may be at heightened risk for suicide. Make sure that your patient understands that this topic is not "off limits," and discuss it openly with them. The following factors (Pope 1986a) may be associated, for some patients, with greater or lesser degrees of suicidal risk: direct statements (always take a suicidal threat or suicidal reference seriously), a formulated plan (the more specific, lethal, and feasible, the higher the risk), past attempts, depression, other clinical syndromes such as organic brain syndrome and schizophrenia, hopelessness, sex, intoxication, age, living alone, bereavement, race, religion, unemployment and/or lack of financial resources, health status, impulsivity, rigid thinking, stressful life events (including but not limited to those mentioned elsewhere in this list), recent release from hospitalization (including brief passes off grounds), and indirect statements and behavioral signs.

Crisis intervention may be necessary, especially during the initial phases of therapy. Develop adequate procedures for working with your patient to handle emergencies. Clarify your availability to your patients. Can you always be reached by phone? Who can they contact in an emergency if you are not available? Handle your absences—both planned (vacations) and unplanned (illness)—with care.

CONDUCT OR ARRANGE FOR A COMPREHENSIVE ASSESSMENT

The effects of the sexual intimacy on the patient's condition need to be examined as fully as permitted by each stage of therapy. The full extent may not become apparent for many years, through long and difficult periods of effort by both patient and therapist. As frequently stressed, patients must be allowed to move at their own pace through this frequently traumatic and terrifying terrain.

Although the sequelae of therapist-patient sexual intimacy may form the heart of the patient's distress and dysfunction, all other factors must be assessed and may need immediate attention. Such areas of inquiry might include, for instance, both current external stressors and long-term personality characteristics.

If a patient has not had a recent comprehensive physical examination, the therapist should recommend one by a qualified physician to rule out possible biological aspects, which may be in need of immediate medical attention. For example, the patient may complain of "tension headaches." These might make sense in terms of the stress caused by the trauma of sexual involvement with a previous therapist, but a variety of organic factors—including a brain tumor—may be involved. An accurate diagnosis should be based upon the best and most comprehensive available data.

In many cases a comprehensive psychological and neuropsychological assessment will play a crucial role in the attempt to arrive at a useful diagnosis and effective treatment plan. The psychologist conducting the assessment must realize that the test protocols and the written report may become evidence in legal or administrative proceedings.

DON'T PRACTICE LAW

There are two crucially important reasons for this prohibition. First, patients who have been sexually intimate with previous therapists may have legal rights to substantial recovery. That is to say, the law respects their right to be made "whole"—insofar as possible—when they have been harmed. The attempt to claim this right, and its interaction with numerous other legal rights and obligations, is exceedingly complex. For example, in filing a suit, they may waive rights to privacy and privilege. There are often statues of limitation, so that delays may waive their rights to recovery. Their filing allied complaints, either concurrently or in sequence, with licensing boards or ethics committees, may affect the probability of prevailing in a malpractice suit. Patients have a right to make their decisions on the basis of expert advice from qualified counsel. In our framework of government, attorneys are those trained and authorized to give such advice. Therapists who try to act as lawyers can compound the damage done by the previous therapist. In the same way that therapists are obligated to have their patients' medical needs assessed and treated by a qualified and licensed physician, they are obligated to have their patients' legal needs be assessed (and a legal courses of action be recommended) by a qualified and duly authorized attorney. Particularly in light of the statutes of limitation, consultation delayed is often consultation denied.

The second reason for the prohibition is that even if the therapist is also an attorney by training, to attempt to serve as both therapist and attorney would involve a dual relationship, a confusion of roles that is likely to be damaging in and of itself for the patient.

ENSURE ACCESS TO INFORMATION CONCERNING THERAPIST-PATIENT SEXUAL INTIMACY

Patients may have been told a number of lies about therapist-patient sexual involvement. They may be unaware that the practice is prohibited by the formal ethical codes of all the major mental health disciplines. They may be unaware that licensing boards can take action against therapists who engage in sexual intimacies with their patients. They may be unaware of the research concerning the practice and its sequelae.

Learning about such issues may play a pivotal role in a patients' coming to grips with an experience in their past that has been, up to this point, shoved out of awareness because it is too painful and overwhelming. Patient education, in this sense, can provide a framework within which patients can begin acknowledging, sorting out, and making sense of their experience.

Many patients are surprised to learn that they are not alone, that others have been through similar experiences. Reading the literature in this area and discussing it with knowledgeable professionals can reduce their sense of isolation and help them deal with feelings of shame, guilt, and confusion.

Some therapists may find it useful to help their patients contact other professionals, third parties who can work with them in the roles of educator and advocate. Such a strategy, as long as it is well-coordinated, can have numerous benefits, one of which is that the patient establishes a number of "connections," and may feel less as if the therapist were his or her only "lifeline." Patients may also find it hard to doubt the aggressive assertions of the previous therapist that therapist-patient sexual intimacy is a legitmate practice and even an integral part of the treatment plan. By talking to a number of independent professionals, as well as by reading the professional literature, patients may become more confident that sexual intimacies between therapists and patients are clinically destructive, legally prohibited, and ethically reprehensible.

RESPECT THE PATIENT'S AUTONOMY

Therapists may feel strongly that a patient "should" either take or refrain from taking action regarding the previous therapist. The therapist may feel that it is best for the patient to put the unpleasant experience in the past "where it belongs" and to get on with life. The therapist may want to avoid becoming involved in protracted legal procedings, to avoid the stress of court appearances, to avoid the wrath and perhaps threats of the former therapist, and so may try to influence the patient to let the entire matter drop. On the other hand, the therapist may want to ensure that no other patients are harmed by the previous therapist. (It should be noted here that many therapists become sexually involved with more than one patient.) Thus the therapist may try to make the patient address a problem that the profession has failed to address adequately. The therapist may simply feel a powerful rage at the offending therapist, and not want to "let him get away with it."

This range of feelings is quite common and understandable. It is the responsibility of the therapist to be aware of these reactions, to handle them responsibly, and to ensure that they do not interfere with the patient's autonomy or with the process of therapy. In all cases it is the patient's right to decide freely, ideally in full knowledge of his or her rights and with access to advice from an attorney, whether to file a civil suit against the former therapist. As noted previously, therapists must refrain from attempting to act as attorneys and from giving bogus legal advice. What therapists can legitimately and therapeutically do is to help patients explore the meaning of the sexual involvement for their life, what their unique needs and wants and goals are, what it might mean for their life and recovery if they were to file a civil suit and if they were to decline filing such a suit. The answers to such questions are neither simple nor readily apparent. The patient's view of the situation may change over the course of therapy. What does not change is the fact that the decision is always and invariably the patient's, not the therapist's. That decision, whatever it is, deserves respect from the therapist.

CONSTRUCT A TREATMENT PLAN SUITED TO THE NEEDS OF THE INDIVIDUAL PATIENT

A number of different modalities of treatment can be effective for patients who have been sexually intimate with their previous therapist. We discuss these approaches in Chapter 8. In some cases the therapist and patient may agree on one specific treatment approach. In other cases the use of several modalities in conjunction with each other seems indicated.

Therapist and patient can discuss the various options, the advantages and drawbacks of each one, and how they might be combined into an effective treatment approach. It will be necessary for both therapist and patient to agree on the treatment plan and to have confidence in it. Patients have a well-established right to give or withhold informed consent to treatment. To ensure that this right is fully exercised, therapists must take steps to see that their patients are fully informed of: the nature of the proposed treatment, the possible liabilities of such treatment as well as the expected benefits, and alternative approaches.

MAINTAIN CLARITY OF ROLES AND COMMUNICATION

Patients who have been sexually intimate with previous therapists may subsequently work with a variety of service-providers. As an example, such a patient may seek subsequent therapy with a social worker. The social worker initiates weekly sessions of individual psychotherapy. He refers the patient to a physician for a comprehensive medical examination, to a psychologist for psychological and neuropsychological assessment, and to a lawyer for legal advice and representation. The patient and social worker decide that individual therapy might be supplemented with group therapy, specifically a group such as the UCLA Post-Therapy Support Group, which provides services to those who have been sexually intimate with their previous therapist. The group is led by cotherapists, a psychiatrist and a psychologist. At this point, the patient is working with six professionals.

Obviously, the necessity for clarity of roles and effective communication among all concerned is central. It is extremely important to recognize that the tasks, backgrounds, and perspectives of the professionals involved may contribute to varying sets of agendas. Additionally, rivalries among the different professions are not unheard of, and professional jealousies, misunderstandings, and "turf issues" are not rare. The professionals involved must handle such potentially destructive factors in such a way that confusion and harm to the patient does not result. They must work actively and responsibly to create an overall structure within which each can do his or her job effectively and both can and will communicate all relevant and appropriate information to the others.

8

Special Principles and Techniques of the Subsequent Therapy

It is difficult to give a specific answer, which fits all cases, to the question: How does the treatment of patients who have been sexually intimate with their former therapists differ from the treatment of other patients? On one hand, patients who have been sexually intimate with their therapists may have been suffering from clinical, developmental, or organic syndromes that originally led them to seek help. These syndromes, such as those described in *DSM-III* (American Psychiatric Association 1980) may afflict any patient, regardless of whether he or she has been sexually involved with a therapist. However, the syndromes may have remained untreated, may have grown substantially worse for lack of appropriate attention, and may have been exacerbated by the sexual intimacies. Further, the expectations about therapy and the ability to form a trusting relationship have been altered, often drastically, by the trauma of the sexualized relationship with the former therapist. Thus, for example, the transference that forms in the subsequent therapy is often extremely intense, ambivalent, and confusing.

Complicating this picture is the fact that therapeutic approaches must fit both the individual therapist and the individual patient. No method is appropriate in all times and places or with all people. However, in our own work and in our study of the field, we have found approaches to the following seven issues to be important and useful:

1. Ambivalence
2. Anger
3. Guilt
4. Depression and Suicide Risk
5. Isolation
6. Sexual Confusion
7. Cognitive Dysfunction

The following sections present approaches to these issues.

AMBIVALENCE

As described earlier in this book, Marmor and others have compared therapist-patient sexual involvement to incest. Both activities often produce an intense ambivalence toward the authority figure who is seen on the one hand as powerful, protective, and even loving, and on the other hand as coldly exploitive. In our society, great trust is placed in therapists, who are charged with providing help to those who are most distressed, needy, vulnerable, and trusting. The state grants special status to therapists, allowing communications to them to be privileged (that is, protected from inquisitive courts). Their testimony as experts in legal proceedings can weigh heavily in such special issues as the placement of children in custody hearings, determinations of someone's accountability for major crimes (for example, in the use of the so-called insanity defense), and the formal abridgement of civil rights (for example, detaining and institutionalizing people against their will by determining them to be "gravely disabled"). It is no wonder, then, that individual patients may look up to and attribute considerable power and prestige to a therapist.

It is more than society's investment of status and prestige onto therapists that influences patients. When they seek help from a therapist, they are likely to project onto that clinician many of their most primitive feelings about a powerful, helping authority. They may come to view the therapist as a savior and a god. The transferring of such feelings (which many of us had as young children about our parents) into the therapeutic situation is common. Most therapists help their patients to become aware of such transference and to handle it therapeutically. In fact, the analysis of the transference is a cornerstone of psychoanalysis and many psychodynamically oriented therapies.

The exploitive therapist tends to nurture and exploit the natural phenomenon of transference. He or she basks in the patient's attention and adoration. Implicitly—sometimes explicitly—the exploitive therapist offers to fulfill the hopes embodied in the transference. All needs will be met. The patient will be taken care of forever by a wise and all-powerful authority. If, as Henry Kissinger once observed, power is the greatest aphrodiasiac, exploitive therapists are in a special position to seduce their patients.

For many patients, their experience with the exploitive therapist is the most powerful of their lives. The sexual experience has been compared to "sleeping with a god." It is no wonder that patients who have been sexually intimate with a former therapists tend to experience a sharp and prolonged ambivalence. They have drawn all the themes of their lives together in the previous therapy and woven them into a single strand of meaning around the exploitive therapist. The protagonists in both *Betrayal* (Freeman and Roy 1976) and *Therapist* (Plaisil 1985) describe vividly just how thorough this process of giving over of the self can be.

Part of the ambivalence may be traced to the energy and force with which such patients have devoted themselves to the therapist. Having invested so much, they can barely consider what it might mean if they have been betrayed. For many, the meaning of their lives has become so deeply identified with their relationship to the exploitive therapist that they can literally not imagine continuing life in any other way.

Another part of the ambivalence may be traced to specific transference. For many patients, the therapist takes on the characteristics of, and in a sense assumes the identity of, some very special person in the patient's earlier life. For example, the patient may come to view the therapist as a father or mother. To recognize that the relationship with the therapist was one of exploitation is to experience "losing" or "giving up" or "being separated from" that earlier special person. The loss is aggravated by the realization that one has been tricked and used.

Yet another part of the ambivalence may be traced to the all-but-inextinguishable hope that somehow, if the patient is truly faithful, the relationship with the former therapist will magically be transformed into what the patient had all along hoped it would be and into what the therapist had, at least implicitly, promised it would be. Thus the ambivalence carrier with it an enormous pressure: the patient fears making "the wrong move." The patient is terrified that, by opening his or her eyes to the reality of the situation, the one chance at eternal love, protection, and happiness will be forfeited forever.

This ambivalence may be confusing, sometimes frightening, to patient and subsequent therapist alike. One moment, the patient acknowledges the exploitive nature of the previous relationship and resolves to work these issues through in the subsequent therapy; the next moment, the patient is convinced that it was all a mistake—due to the patient's stupidity and lack of trust—and resolves to return to the exploitive therapist to beg for forgiveness and to be taken back. These "swings" can be unexpected, sudden, and forceful.

Such ambivalence is sometimes resolved early in the subsequent therapy, but in our experience this is relatively rare. In most instances it seems to take a long time and great effort and tenacity for patients to work through these extremely deep contradictory feelings. Their appearance in the middle and later stages of the subsequent therapy can pose a special threat to the patient's recovery for they engender disappointment and sometimes despair. The patient thinks: "I have worked so long and so hard, and I thought I had resolved all that, but here I am thinking that maybe I did the wrong thing by leaving him after all."

As is the case with many of these intense thoughts and feelings, the subsequent therapist's patience, acceptance, and confidence (in the patient and in the process of the subsequent therapy) are crucial. If the subsequent therapist communicates—either directly or indirectly—fear, disgust, or other negative reactions to the patient's ambivalence, the patient is likely to feel that the ambivalence is taboo. The patient will then keep silent about these feelings, acting (with the subsequent therapist) as if the ambivalence is not present. Driven underground, the ambivalence is not available for exploration and therapeutic resolution. The patient is likely to feel shame and disgust at thinking "such vile thoughts." Premature termination may be one result of not being able to deal with the ambivalence in the subsequent therapy. In extreme cases, the patient may be so tortured and confused by the chronic and persistent nature of this taboo feeling that he or she will attempt to get rid of it by the only means that seem available: suicide.

If the ambivalence is deeply rooted, it is likely that the patient will experience it as part of the transference toward the subsequent therapist. For example, a patient may feel ambivalent toward the exploitive therapist. Part of the time she desires to be rid of that therapist and of the painful and destructive experience that constituted that relationship. But at other times she desperately wants to re-create the intimacy she felt with him. At any cost, she wishes to return to him and to fulfill the implicit promises he made to her. In her subsequent therapy she may experience at times a sudden desire to abandon the subsequent therapist, to be rid of him at all costs. At other times she may feel a desire to establish with him the same sort of relationship she had with the previous therapist. Thus she may feel a need for psychological and physical merging, including sexual intimacy.

When patients experience this sort of ambivalence as part of the transference to their subsequent therapist, explicit reassurance in two areas is particularly helpful to them. First, the subsequent therapist can assure them that such feelings are a natural response in light of their previous experience. They will be treated with acceptance and respect. The therapist can stress that he or she will help the patient to explore these feelings. Second, the therapist can assure them that under no circumstances will the patient's desire for sexual contact be acted out within the therapy. It is crucial that this reassurance be done in such a way that does not encourage the patient to feel guilty or ashamed about having experienced or verbally expressed the feelings.

Because the previous therapy may have included many indirect communications and implicit promises, it may be important in the subsequent therapy for the therapist to take sufficient time to discuss such issues openly, specifically, and clearly. If, for example, the patient says that some of the time she wishes she could make love with the subsequent therapist, and if the therapist does not provide an explicit reassurance that this will not occur under any conditions, the patient may fantasize that, perhaps as in the previous therapy, sexual union will be an eventual occurrence. Such an unaddressed fantasy may become so frightening to the patient that is may lead to the patient's failure to discuss related issues in the therapy and perhaps to the patient's premature termination of therapy as an understandably defensive measure.

ANGER

Patients often experience an intense anger toward a previous therapist with whom they have been sexually involved. So intense is this anger that it may threaten to overwhelm the patient and, in some cases, the subsequent therapist.

The anger is understandable. The patient, hurting and vulnerable, sought help from the former therapist and was given instead an enormously damaging "treatment." The patient feels cheated, the victim of an outrageously fradulent act. The therapist had set aside the customary stance of attempting to be of help to the patient and had, instead, met his or her own needs using the patient as the instrument of satisfaction. Thus the patient did not get what is normally offered in therapy, did not get legitimate treatment. This offense may strike the patient as even more intolerable in light of the fact that the patient (or the patient's insurance company, or the patient's spouse or parents) paid the exploitive therapist for the sessions of sex.

The wound goes deeper, however. It is not only that the exploitive therapist failed to deliver the customary clinical services, but also that he or she failed to keep the implicit promises to deliver more magical services (related to the transference) as described in the previous section on ambivalence. The patient, in collusion with the therapist, may have fantasized that the therapist was in a position to deliver all sorts of wonderful blessings, none of which ever will be forthcoming. The more primitive the patient's wants and needs that the therapist utilizes in the seduction, the more destructive the process and the more intense the rage that later emerges.

Thus the patient feels betrayed on two levels: the realistic and the more deeply subjective. The sometimes gradual realization that he or she will not receive fulfillment of either rational or irrational expectations that were encouraged by the previous therapist can fill a patient with rage.

The rage can intensify as the patient comes to grips with the fact that the exploitive therapist not only will not honor his or her promises, but also never intended to honor them. The previous "therapy" seems to the patient more and more a charade in which the patient was tricked, lied to, and used.

This anger is often repressed or suppressed by the patient, and is not infrequently turned against oneself. It may then be experienced as guilt, as depression, and sometimes as an impulse to commit suicide.

Often the previous therapist may have taught the patient to suppress or rechannel such anger. Few exploitive therapists will tolerate their patients expressing anger toward them. Sometimes they will direct the patient to redefine or relabel the anger as something else. Thus patients who have been sexually involved with previous therapists may be quite confused about their own feelings. They have learned to screen them out or to pretend they are something else. Sometimes exploitive therapists will tell their patients that anger felt toward the therapist is a sign that there is something wrong with the patient. Plasil (1985) drew a vivid picture of a therapist who could tolerate neither anger nor disagreement, who would explain that there must be something wrong with a patient who would be angry at such a kind and perfect therapist.

Subsequent therapists, therefore, may have to provide considerable reassurance to their patients that the experience and verbal expression of anger are a natural occurrence and can be important parts of the therapeutic process. Such anger can be reflected in the transference to the subsequent therapist, and patients need to be reassured that this, too, is understandable and a part of the therapeutic process. Even with such reassurances, patients may fear that their anger, once expressed, will either be so powerful that it will somehow destroy the therapist or be so offensive that the subsequent therapist will punish them (perhaps by terminating the therapy or labeling them as "crazy").

The fact that patients may experience anger toward the subsequent therapist as part of the transference does not mean that they can never feel more rationally based anger toward that therapist. All of us are human, and from time to time we will make errors in judgment, giving our clients quite legitimate grounds for anger. Acknowledgement of such errors and of the hurt and anger they cause is an important aspect of any honest therapy. Since the patients who are the subject of this book are often prone to self-doubt and to an impaired sensitivity to their own feelings and perceptions and often have difficulty expressing their anger, it is crucial to take a patient's expression of anger at the subsequent therapist as the starting point of an open exploration. Patients can learn self-awareness and self-trust by this process of exploration.

Thus a patient's anger toward a subsequent therapist may represent transference from the previous "therapy" (or any previous experience) or it may represent an undistorted reaction to actual events in the current therapy. Or it may have elements of both. Whatever conclusions the patient reaches as to the nature of such angry feelings, the process of exploration is therapeutic.

In cases when the patient's anger seems a clear, undistorted reaction to events within the session such as therapist errors, the patient's expression of the anger and the therapist's open acknowledgement of the mistake carry an added benefit. The patient, through this concrete form of reality testing, gains first-hand experience that therapists are, after all, only human. They are not perfect. Even when well-intentioned and scrupulous about their work, they make mistakes. This realization may help the patient to deal with both the idealization of the previous therapist and a generalized tendency to idealize authority figures.

Once therapy becomes a safe place in which to acknowledge and deal with anger and rage, there will be less need for the patient to suppress or repress such feelings. Thus there will be less cause to act them out, as the only way of expressing them (while keeping them out of awareness). There will be also less tendency to turn the negative feelings against oneself as the only permissible channel of expression.

GUILT

Guilt, often interlaced with shame, can be an anguishing experience for patients who have been sexually involved with a therapist. For some, the guilt is predominantly in the sexual area. Many report long-standing sexual problems and concerns. Sometimes these issues prompted the patient to seek help from a professional in the first place. For these patients the disastrous experience of sexual involvement with a therapist is the most dramatic and enduring confirmation that their sexuality is "bad." They tell us: "See, I knew my sexuality would get me into trouble."

For others, the guilt focuses on the exploitive therapist's oft-repeated assertion: "The patient started it!" Such therapists seek to evade any responsibility for their failure to uphold sound clinical, ethical, and legal standards by claiming helplessness vis-a-vis the patient's intense needs or subtle wiles. It is not unlike the rapist's stance of blaming it on the seductive clothing of the victim or the incest perpetrator's claim that a child was ir- resistably inviting. Patients who have been sexually involved with their therapist are often, because of their tendency to be self-critical, very vulnerable to such outrageous claims.

Unfortunately, our culture may show some tendency to "blame the vic- tim" and thus unfortunately support the "don't blame me, blame the patient!" charges of exploitive therapists. Most readers of this book will have little trouble remembering court cases in which rape charges were dismissed on the basis of such factors as the victim's clothing. On July 9, 1985, a veteran judge "ruled that an 8-year-old girl consented to sexual acts and then reduced rape charges against the two men [her uncle and her mother's boyfriend] ac- cused of assaulting her" (L.A. *Times*, 1985, p. A-6). However, a gradual but steady change has been occurring in our cultural climate. The tendency to blame the victim of a sexual, assaultive, or exploitive act has diminished, in- itially in regard to such behaviors as rape, incest, and spouse battering, and more recently in regard to therapist-patient sexual intimacy.

For still others, guilt focuses primarily on the termination of the relationship with the previous therapist, speaking to someone else (such as a subsequent therapist), or perhaps filing formal charges against the perpetrator. Patients have attributed such qualities and powers to the therapists with whom they've been sexually involved that failing to obey the therapist's wishes seems an act of heresy. For many, it is not unlike going against the will of God. The guilt is enormous. It may be compared to the guilt felt by a child who tells someone about the "secret" relationship with an incestuous parent.

Exploitive therapists work hard at laying the groundwork for such guilt to protect the secrecy of their illicit acts. They stress, in the therapy sessions, how helpless and needy the patient is, and how much the therapist has skillfully, generously provided help. The exploitive therapist feels more secure when the patient is saddled with an oppressive sense of indebtedness.

When a patient seems to be slipping out of the psychological grasp of the exploitive therapist, new measures are taken. The therapist, knowing the vulnerabilities of the individual patient, will describe the terrible consequences (for the therapist) should the patient report the offense. The therapist will lose the license to practice and thus lose income. The therapist's spouse will sue for divorce. Colleagues and friends will shun the therapist. He or she will be vilified by the media, who "don't understand this special relationship." The therapist's health, already failing, will be dealt a devastating blow. The therapist will commit suicide. Can the patient tolerate the guilt of "causing" all this to happen to someone with whom he or she was intimate?

As with so many areas of communication between therapists and patients who are sexually involved, the therapist's messages are often inconsistent. Such claims of vulnerability to the patient's revelations are not infrequently alternated with the therapist's claims that: (1) the patient is crazy and has imagined the whole thing, (2) no one will believe the patient, or if they do, they won't care or do anything about it, (3) the therapist can have the patient committed, or drugged, or lobotomized, or (4) the therapist can arrange for the patient (or one of the patient's family members) to "meet with an accident." Since the patient has been attributing such power and authority to the therapist, such threats tend to carry great weight. Paradoxically, the more confusing and inconsistent the statements, the more powerful they are, for the patient has more trouble thinking them through clearly and determining their validity.

The guilt that patients carry with them from their relationship with an exploitive therapist tends to have an oppressive and paralyzing effect. It is important that the subsequent therapists not refuse to hear the patient's expression of such feelings. However well intentioned, attempts to dismiss the patient's feelings will produce an "echo" of the previous therapy (in which the patient's feelings were not respected) and the patient will not feel "heard." The patient and subsequent therapist can work together to explore such feelings and to work them through. In some cases the patient will benefit from objective information (for example, that the previous therapist has no power to lobotomize the patient). In other cases the patient will benefit from a chance to explore the ways in which long-standing guilt feelings—some perhaps from early childhood—were augmented, manipulated, and distorted through the efforts of the previous therapist. It may be that guilt feelings were one of the reasons the patient originally sought therapy. Such feelings may be openly and therapeutically addressed, once the harm from the relationship with the previous therapist has been sufficiently lessened.

DEPRESSION AND SUICIDE RISK

In our experience, the most common presenting complaint of patients who have been sexually intimate with a previous therapist is depression. Perhaps the most central aspect of this depression is the intense sense of loss. In almost all cases, the transference in regard to the previous therapist has been substantial. The patient had developed an extremely idealized view of and attachment to the therapist. As mentioned previously, the therapist who develops a sexually intimate relationship with a patient becomes like god, a parent (as seen through the eyes of a very young child), an omniscient and almost omnipotent authority figure. The patient starts to focus his or her whole life on this persona, and develops a strong dependence.

Then this idealized persona and relationship are lost. It is important to stress that the loss includes all of the patient's expectations—which were subtly or directly encouraged by the therapist.

Originally the patient went to the therapist for help, for treatment. As Freud asserted, and as subsequent experience and research have borne out, once the sexual contact begins, the treatment ends. So the patient has lost the help that was originally expected.

Furthermore, the patient has lost the idealized persona and relationship, along with all the expectations that were a part of them. Because the attachment to the therapist was so profound and intense, many patients feel as if life no longer has any meaning.

The experience of this loss—both of the original hope for treatment and of the idealized persons and relationship—can precipitate a devastating depression. It is all the more difficult for the patient to deal with because the former attempt to get help for a psychological problem turned out to be so destructive. Thus the patient is extremely reluctant to make further efforts to get help.

In light of the intensity of the depression, the increased risk of suicide is understandable. The ambivalence (making it hard for patients to think clearly about their situation and the causes of the depression), the guilt (reinforcing the sense that the misery they are experiencing is their own fault), and the anger (which is so often turned inward upon the self) all tend to interact in such a way as to make suicide seem the best—the only—option.

The exploitive therapist may be quite aware of the incipient depression and suicidal tendencies and may actually try to augment them. Some therapists have actively urged or commanded their patients to commit suicide as a preventive measure to ensure that no third parties find out about the sexual intimacies.

In some cases the depression may be masked or otherwise not readily apparent. Many patients, in order to continue living what has become an excruciatingly painful life, have made full use of such defenses as denial and reaction formation. "Smiling compliance" and "smiling depression" are thus not uncommon.

Whether or not depression is one of the presenting complaints when the patient seeks help with a subsequent therapist, depression often emerges during the course of the subsequent therapy and requires considerable therapeutic work.

The depression may intensify during the course of the subsequent therapy as the patient becomes more and more able to acknowledge and explore the relationship with the previous therapist. It is important for the patient to feel, as much as possible, "in control" of the pace of such therapeutic work. That is to say, it is generally unhelpful (and sometimes quite contratherapeutic) for the therapist to "push" the patient to explore areas for which the patient is not ready.

Developing an effective working alliance with a patient may be quite difficult in this regard. The patient may always have felt out of control in the previous therapy. Thus it is hard for the patient to trust the new therapist and to learn to trust his or her own impulses as to what can be explored safely and therapeutically during any given session. Open discussion between therapist and patient of the difficulties of forming an effective working alliance and other such "process" issues can be very beneficial.

Enabling the patient to feel more in control of the content and pace of the sessions does not, of course, mean that the therapist is passive. What it does mean is that the therapist neither blocks the patient from exploring a given area of experience, no matter how painful, nor coerces the patient into discussing a topic for which the patient is not ready. The therapist must actively and continuously assess the patient's condition, particularly with regard to serious depression and suicidal risk. When depression threatens to overwhelm the patient and makes suicide a possibility, the therapist must work actively with the patient to ensure that there are adequate measures taken to ensure the patient's safety and well-being. Therapists should not hesitate to ask the patient directly if the feelings of depression seem overwhelming, out of control, or threatening to elicit self-destructive behavior.

ISOLATION

If the patient has experienced the previous therapist as an omniscient, omnipotent "significant other" and this relationship is now lost, it is not surprising that the patient may now feel alone in the world and isolated. Many feel—initially at least—that their relationship to the previous therapist was unique and that no one else could possibly understand their experience. Thus they feel isolated on two levels. First, they are isolated in the world, separated from the person who had given meaning to their life. Second, they are isolated from any understanding of their personal experience and situation; it is difficult for them to believe that the subsequent therapist or anyone else could offer them genuine understanding and empathy.

It is crucial, then, for the subsequent therapist to establish, insofar as possible, a sense of rapport with the patient and to communicate empathy effectively. The difficulty of this task and its inherent frustrations may be disconcerting for the therapist and may elicit a variety of countertransferential reactions. The patient may mistrust the therapist's expressions of care and concern and may resist them vigorously. A major danger is that the therapist, experiencing no acceptance or even acknowledgement of attempts to offer support and caring, may withdraw and contribute to the patient's experience of isolation. The subsequent therapist may also experience impulses to withdraw if the patient's intense neediness to be "connected" (to counteract the feelings of isolation) seems overwhelming, draining, or frightening.

Symptoms of the therapist's attempts to disengage from the patient are varied, and the effective therapist is alert for them. The therapist may find him- or herself "forgetting," canceling (with inadequate cause), or reducing the frequency (without basing the reduction on the clinical needs of the patient) the patient's appointments. Between sessions the therapist may experience dread of the next appointment. During sessions the therapist may experience prolonged boredom, daydreaming (about topics essentially unrelated to the therapy, or perhaps about transferring the patient to another therapist), or eagerness for the session to be over. Such countertransferential reactions are, of course, relevant to the therapy. It is crucial that the therapist be aware of any such reactions and explore adequately their implications for effective work with the patient.

Some exploitive therapists attempt to isolate their patients. They do not refer them for medical examinations (even if the patient complains of physical symptoms), for psychological testing (even if this would be clinically useful), for an independent interview and "second opinion," for adjunctive therapeutic modalities, and so on. Furthermore, the therapist may encourage or command the patient to break off relationships with friends and relatives, particularly spouses. This strategy of isolation accomplishes two objectives. First, by minimizing the patient's contacts with third parties, the therapist minimizes the possibility that the secret (the sexual relationship between therapist and patient) will be disclosed. Second, by cutting the patient off from other resources, the therapist becomes a relatively more important—perhaps crucial—lifeline for the patient's continued functioning.

In light of the isolation experienced by so many patients who have been sexually intimate with the previous therapist, it is important to work with them to counteract this isolation. Thus scheduling an independent medical examination, a psychological and neuropsychological assessment, an interview with a colleague who can provide the patient with a "second opinion," and other such procedures can not only fulfil their customary clinical functions but can also provide direct benefit to the patient who will have less reason to regard the subsequent therapist as his or her only lifeline. Such procedures can be particularly helpful when—as often happens—the transference to the subsequent therapist is intense.

SEXUAL CONFUSION

The trauma of sexual intimacies with a therapist often affects the patient's understanding of sexuality, sense of him- or herself as a sexual being, and sexual behavior.

Some patients develop an almost phobic avoidance of sexual relationships and activity. This aspect of their lives has become infused with a confusing sense of horror, guilt, betrayal, and sadness. For many of those who have developed posttraumatic stress disorder, any reminder of sexuality or sexual behavior is likely to evoke traumatic flashbacks, nightmares, intrusive thoughts, or unbidden images. In extreme cases, a psychotic break can be precipitated.

Other patients develop compulsive sexual behavior. In some cases this can be viewed as an attempt to re-create the intimacy that was experienced with the previous therapist. In other cases it may be the result of the previous therapist's urgings or commands that the patient engage in promiscuous sexual behavior or behaviors of certain types preferred by the therapist. Such urgings and commands have been generally accepted unquestioningly by the patient, even long after the sessions with the previous therapist have been discontinued. Frequently, such compulsive behavior subsequently occasions deep depression as well as shame and guilt for the patient. Suicide may appear to the patient to be the only method by which such compulsive behavior can be stopped. Secondary damage in such cases of compulsive sexual behavior can occur in the form of sexually transmitted diseases, unwanted pregnancies, and dangerous situations (for example, when the therapist has asserted that the sex must include violence or occur with strangers).

For some patients, sexual difficulties were the presenting problem in the former therapy. Dysfunctions as varied as disorders of sexual desire or arousal, inability to experience orgasm, premature ejaculation, vaginismus, and dyspareunia may have brought the patient to seek professional help originally. Such conditions are almost invariably made worse by sexual involvement with the therapist.

In some cases the trauma has been so profound that the patient has difficulty accurately distinguishing sexual impulses, sensations, or feelings from affects or other experiences. Thus a patient who becomes extremely angry or anxious may label the experience as "sexual arousal." Situational cues that seem to the patient to have nothing to do with sex may elicit sexual fantasies, impulses, arousal, or behavior. Such reactions may be part of the patient's more general feelings of being "out of control."

These sexual issues may be very hard for the patient to explore in the subsequent therapy (and thus elicit resistance), especially in light of the fear, shame, guilt, and disgust they often evoke. Furthermore, sexual feelings may be a significant part of the transference to the subsequent therapist, further complicating the situation.

Perhaps the first and most crucial step in creating a therapeutic environment in which these issues can be explored and resolved is to assure the patient that the therapeutic setting is safe. The therapist should not hesitate to make explicit that he or she will not engage in sexual contact with the patient. This kind of reassurance may need to be repeated frequently as the therapy progresses. As mentioned previously, it is important that this reassurance be offered in a way that does not evoke shame or guilt on the part of the patient. Given that the patient may have felt out of control in the previous therapy and may currently feel out of control, the therapist's clear assurance that no sexual intimacies will occur can help a patient to explore more openly and less defensively his or her own sexual thoughts, feelings, fantasies, and impulses.

Second, ask the patient if there are any steps that could be taken that would help the patient to feel more safe in the therapeutic environment. Some patients, for instance, find any physical contact with the subsequent therapist—no matter how well-intended—sexually arousing or threatening. Thus explicit ground rules can include the stipulation that the therapist and patient will not touch each other. Such ground rules can produce a number of benefits. They can create an environment in which patient and therapist can work together most effectively. They communicate a respect for the patient's wants and needs, a respect that was lacking in the previous therapy. They demonstrate that sexual issues can be discussed openly. Like the treatment plan itself, such ground rules may be augmented and revised as the therapy progresses.

Third, assure the patient that while the therapeutic situation and relationship prohibit sexual intimacy between therapist and patient, the patient need not censor any thoughts, feelings, fantasies, impulses, or other material. Especially in the area of sex, patients are often so ashamed and mistrustful of their own cognitions and affects that they believe this area to be taboo. Certain thoughts seem too horrible, fantasies too shameful, impulses too dirty, to acknowledge and explore, even in the seemingly safe context of therapy. The patient's lack of trust in the therapeutic situation is understandable, of course, in light of the inappropriate and destructive ways in which sexual issues were handled in the previous therapy. Thus many patients fear that if they discuss sexual issues frankly—without censorship, euphemism, or circumlocution—the subsequent therapist will either use the discussion as an opportunity to seduce the patient, or respond in an angry, judgmental, and critical manner at the patient's "shameful attempt to talk dirty." Especially if the transference involves sexual aspects, patients may fear that the subsequent therapist will view them as seductive and will place the blame for what happened to the patient in the previous therapy squarely on the shoulders of the patient.

The patient's view of the subsequent therapist as angry, judgmental, or critical may be a significant aspect of the transference. The previous therapist (and perhaps the patient's parent if incest is a salient issue) may have exploited the patient sexually. But the sexual contact may have been expressed in the context of the previous therapist's shame, guilt, and disgust at sexuality (perhaps related to a sexual dysfunction on the part of the therapist), of sexually infused rage against people of a particular gender, race, or sexual orientation, or of more complex sexual conflicts. Thus the previous therapist may have conveyed contempt for the patient's sexuality and sexual behavior while engaging the patient in a sexual relationship.

If the transference does involve the patient viewing the subsequent therapist as a cold, angry, rejecting authority where sexual issues are concerned, it may be some time before the patient is ready to acknowledge this fact. It may be far into the therapy before the patient discusses how he or she tried to avoid the therapist's wrath by dressing in "approved" ways, avoiding certain make-up, sitting in an awkward position, adopting a stilted and abstract manner of speech, expressing views that would likely not provoke criticism from the therapist, and avoiding all mention of sexuality.

The transference can be quite intense. Some patients are afraid that they will be called "whores" or "sluts" if they wear dresses (rather than bulky slacks) or if they fail to sit awkwardly on the edge of the chair or couch ("like a lady"). Even if the therapist offer frequent assurances that there is no "dress code" or "correct way of sitting" in therapy, the patient may suspect that the therapist secretly condemns the patient.

In such situations, the subsequent therapist has—through the transference—assumed the role of powerful adult or even god. Clarifying through open and, if necessary, frequent discussion that the therapist is not there to tell the patient how to think, feel, dress, sit, or talk is important. Patients may have a difficult time conceptualizing, accepting, and feeling comfortable in a working relationship—in which the therapist does not control the life of the patient and the patient controls his or her own life—that is so different from the one into which they were indoctrinated in their previous therapy.

Fourth, while assuring the patient that any words or ideas may be expressed in therapy, the therapist must make it clear to the patient that there will be no coercion to discuss certain areas. For most patients, therapy is a progression through stages. They may not, for example, be ready to discuss certain thoughts or feelings—in the realm of sexuality or any other realm—for weeks, months, or perhaps years. To try to force a premature discussion of issues such as sexuality for which the client is not ready can seriously compound the damage done by the previous therapist. During any given session, patients should feel confident that they are free to discuss—in full and frank detail—a given subject, but that they are also free not to address that subject. The choice is theirs.

In summary, the therapist must communicate genuine caring and respect for the patient and for the patient's thoughts, feelings, impulses, fantasies, behavior, and choices. This is an active rather than a passive stance, though it does not involve attempts by the therapist to control the patient, either by pushing the patient to discuss material that the patient does not want to discuss (at least at the present time) or by establishing taboo areas of material that the patient is forbidden to explore and address therapeutically.

COGNITIVE DYSFUNCTION

Patients who have been sexually intimate with a previous therapist often experience cognitive dysfunction. Attention and concentration are sometimes impaired. The general difficulties of cognitive functioning are often related to more specific cognitions that are extremely disruptive and over which the patient feels little if any control. Among the most common are flashbacks (related to the previous therapist), nightmares, unbidden thoughts, and intrusive images. Such phenomena are characteristic of post-traumatic stress disorder.

The disruption caused by these cognitions can be extensive and devastating. The impairment of such fundamental processes as attention and cognition can lead to inability to maintain a job or to take care of day-to-day activities. However, the phenomenological aspects are equally destructive. At the mercy of flashbacks, nightmares, and related "uncontrolled" phenomena, the patients come to experience their inner environment (that is, their private world) as painful, threatening, and unpredictable. It is worth noting here that posttraumatic stress disorder is generally considered to be more severe and long-lasting when the stressor is of human agency (Horowitz 1984, p. 373), which of course it is in cases of therapist-patient sexual intimacy.

For many patients the first step is to help them gain some initial control over and relief from the frightening and "out of control" cognitions. Cognitive-behavioral technique are often helpful in this regard. Cautela and McCullough (1978), for example, present procedures for "thought stopping." Beck (1970) demonstrated how a patient with intrusive images could learn to stop these images by clapping his hands.

Second, an overall framework for therapy should be discussed and agreed upon by both therapist and patient. In cases in which there are disruptive cognitions, the diagnosis of posttraumatic stress disorder should be seriously considered. Horowitz (1984, pp. 374–375) outlines a common treatment approach for PTSD:

> Psychotherapy should begin with reconstruction and review of the past, move on to present difficulties, and conclude when adaptive mechanisms for future use are in an adequate state of recovery. . . . Posttraumatic stress disorder may itself modify the personality, so that in chronic cases that come to therapy there is much to be done after dealing with the reaction to the stressful event itself.

As mentioned previously under the section devoted to "Sexual Confusion," the patient should never be coerced to deal with material for which he or she is not ready. Such coercion may lead to a psychotic break, the emergence of uncontrollable suicidal impulses, or other destructive consequences. Especially during the early and middle stages of therapy, the patient needs to maintain adequate relief from the trauma, even as he or she attempts to come to grips with it. Horowitz (1984, p. 374) emphasizes that among the first therapeutic priorities is to ease the strain and put the victim at rest for as long as necessary and by whatever means may be necessary. During the period of protection from strain, the victim may slowly come to acknowledge and tolerate aspects of the experience that were denied before. In chronic post-traumatic stress disorder, this resource is usually not available. Denial is sometimes a normal regulating mechanism that adjusts the amount of unpleasantness perceived to a tolerable level. This necessary process of denial must be respected even as it is addressed therapeutically.

Third, those aspects of the trauma that have previously gained expression through unbidden thoughts, intrusive images, flashbacks, nightmares, and such, must be gradually acknowledged and worked through. These aspects have been too painful and overwhelming for the patient's ordinary conscious awareness. Thus they are repressed, denied, and/or suppressed. Yet they are so powerful that they break into awareness in fragmented and frightening form. Because these aspects have not been processed and integrated into the patient's awareness, they remain out of control and alien. They are like a stuck record that continues to repeat the same passage.

A similar process may happen to any of us on a less intense level. For example, we may have been sitting at a traffic light, daydreaming while waiting for the light to change. Suddenly there is a squeal of tires, a bang of metal, and we feel the jolt as someone smashes into us. Perhaps no one is hurt and the damage to the cars is slight. Nonetheless, most people would experience this as a minor trauma. For the next few days, we may jump at the slightest noise. We may reexperience the wreck in our nightmares. Unbidden images of the accident may intrude into our awareness, causing us to relive the event as if it were happening in the present.

This process, in a much deeper, more complex, and destructive manner, is experienced by the person who experiences cognitive dysfunction as a result of a sexual relationship with a therapist. The concept of reliving the event as if it were happening in the present is central. Discussing post-traumatic stress disorder, Horowitz (1984, p. 374) noted:

> The vicim's mental catalogue of life experiences must be expanded to accommodate the traumatic event. Until this adjustment has been made, the victim's "memory" of the traumatic event retains in the present what belongs in the past even after the immediate strain is over. Reliving the event maintains the supply of intrusive ideas and feelings whether the victim is awake or asleep. Efforts to avoid such painful experiences lead to narrowing of interests, worsening of the quality of life, and formation of other symptoms such as denial numbing. Phases of denial may alternate with periods of intrusion as the patient works through the stress and eventually completes the stress cycle.

Likewise, Scrignar (1984, p. 24) wrote that "the covert encephalic activity of thinking, visualizing, and elaborating on various elements of the traumatic incident keeps the trauma fresh and alive, and plays a major role in the maintenance of a PTSD." This insistent material from the past may alter the patient's cognitions in extreme ways. Horowitz (1984, p. 374) described dissociative states that "may last for minutes to hours or even days. During dissociative states, victims may act as if they are reliving the event."

The therapeutic phase of "reconstruction and review of the past" may be aided by the use of imagery and other cognitive-behavioral techniques that deal directly with the unbidden thoughts, intrusive images, flashbacks, nightmares, and related cognitions (Horowitz 1976, 1978a, 1978b; Meichenbaum 1978; J. L. Singer 1974; Singer and Pope 1978; Pope 1982, 1985a, 1985b; Levenson and Pope 1984). These methods give patients a safe and supportive framework for attending carefully to the images, exploring them in detail in an unhurried manner, and integrating them into the patients' more general experience and understanding.

Patience on the part of the therapist is crucial to this work. A single image—perhaps a terrifying flashback to an incident with the previous therapist—can be so overwhelming for the patient that several sessions may be needed to explore it. Even after it seems to have been well integrated into the patient's experience, it may return unexpectedly in subsequent stages of therapy, indicating that there are still unresolved issues to be addressed.

This reconstruction and review can take place only once some initial relief has been gained by the patient and once the cognitions seem less overwhelmingly threatening, more manageable. Thus the various thought-stopping techniques are "first aid" rather than final treatment. They give the patient initial relief from the terror and pain of the cognitions and help the patient to develop a sense of control over these mental processes. They help enable the patient to approach the work of reconstruction and review.

Some severely dysfunctional patients, especially in the intial and middle phases of treatment, may find the periods between sessions very difficult to tolerate. They may not yet have developed the ability to cope effectively with the unbidden images, flashbacks, and intrusive thoughts that become overwhelming. Specific procedures may be implemented to help them lessen the pain and anxiety of these intersession periods while engaging in therapeutic work.

For example, some patients (Pope 1985a) find it helpful to spend perhaps an hour a day reviewing and working through the cognitions using a tape recorder or notebook. They may then bring the tapes or notebooks to the therapy sessions for review, or simply discuss the content. Such an approach has several potential advantages:

1. It encourages a more active stance on the part of a patient who may

feel helpless vis-a-vis the negative mental images, and who may have been indoctrinated (by the former therapist) into a passive stance vis-a-vis a therapist. It stresses the patient's active initiative and involvement in the recovery process.

2. It helps the patient to structure time and activities. Patients who are unable to work or otherwise carry on ordinary daily activities often find themselves in a downward spiral of depression and anxiety. The patient can now schedule a daily activity that is of obvious importance, and that the patient may carry out independently. The out-of-control cognitions can often have an insistent quality. They drag the patient's awareness into revery, obsessive thinking, or dissociative states. They are healthy in that they signal an awareness that there is important material that has not been sufficiently attended to and integrated into the patient's life. Attempts to steadfastly ignore these cognitions between sessions are often futile. However, if the patient is assured of a specific time each day when the attention will be devoted exclusively to these cognitions, he or she can more easily spend the rest of the day on other activities without the intrusion of such cognitions and without the sense that there is incomplete work constantly pressing for attention.

3. It helps the patient to internalize the process of therapy. For extremely needy patients, the tape recorder itself or the notebook can serve as transitional objects, helping the patient to learn to tolerate the absence of the therapist. It can help symbolize and implement the patient's increasing independence from the therapist.

4. It helps the patient to begin translating the images into words, which facilitates the process of understanding and integration (Horowitz 1976, 1978a, 1978b; Meichenbaum 1978; Singer and Pope 1978).

Therapists whose primary orientation is psychoanalytic or psychodynamic may have reservations concerning whether such cognitive-behavioral methods can be effectively integrated into their own approach. There is, however, evidence that the blending of the two can be effective (Levenson and Pope 1984).

The issues and methods presented in this chapter have been useful in helping patients who have been sexually intimate with a previous therapist. It is important to note, however, that only in the last two decades have the mental health professions engaged in the serious and systematic study of therapist-patient sexual intimacy, the damage it causes, and treatment for the harmed patients. In terms of developing clearly conceptualized, effective, and efficient treatment approaches, we are just beginning.

9

Problems and Prospects for Patients Filing Complaints

Chapters 9, 10, and 11 focus on the formal complaint process itself, from the perspectives first of patients (the present chapter), then of attorneys (Chapter 10), and finally of professionals who serve as expert witnesses (Chapter 11).

This chapter is addressed specifically to patients, though it may be of use to therapists, attorneys, consultants, advocates, and anyone attempting to be of help to patients who are considering filing a formal complaint against a therapist.

It is our opinion, based on our own clinical experience and our review of the literature in this area, that filing a complaint with a civil court, a licensing board, or a professional ethics committee can be an important, positive, and healing experience for patients who have been sexually involved with their therapists. It can be a constructive assertion of one's rights, helping to counteract feelings of passive victimization. It can be a formal acknowledgement of the reality of what has happened, part of the necessary process of working through a trauma. It can be part of the process of reemergence into the community of family and friends, breaking the bonds of silence and secrecy imposed by the therapist. It can be means by which a consumer holds accountable the professional for his or her violation of professional standards. It can be an act of considerable altruism, motivated by the desire to see that the professional is prevented from engaging in such acts with other patients. It can be an act of courage and self-affirmation, a refusal to be intimidated into paralysis by the explicit and implicit threats of the exploitive therapist.

We believe that it "can be" one or more of these positive steps but that some patients may choose not to press any formal charges and that, for them, this is the right choice. Some may feel themselves too fragile and vulnerable, too devastated and preoccupied with simply "holding on" to take on the rigors of filing a complaint. Others may value their privacy more than any possible gains from the complaint process. Still others may decide that the realities of the complaint systems available to them in their own personal situation simply can not be trusted to provide an acceptable outcome. It is important to note here that the investment of time and energy required to file and follow up on a complaint in the malpractice courts, the administrative law system, and, in most cases, professional ethics committees is considerable, often lasting years. Patients must remain constantly aware of this fact as they decide whether or not to pursue one or more formal complaints.

It is crucial for patients to recognize that the choice is always theirs. The people around them may, consciously or unwittingly, urge them either to file or not to file, but the decision correctly and ultimately belongs to the patient.

The best decisions in this regard are made not in haste, but after careful deliberation. They are based upon information that is as complete and accurate as possible. They are the result of self-exploration, and awareness of one's wants, needs, values, and resources. Not infrequently, consultation with a variety of trusted individuals plays an important role.

The decision whether to file or not to file is a deeply personal one. The avenues to the final decision are as varied as the individuals facing this dilemma. However, the issues discussed in the following sections may be of help to those who are considering options regarding the filing of formal complaints.

RECOGNIZE YOUR OWN REACTIONS

Recognize the many profound and sometimes conflicting reactions you may be having to your relationship with the exploitive therapist. Some of the reactions that are frequently reported by those who have been sexually intimate with their therapists are discussed in this book, particularly in Chapters 5 and 8.

These reactions may be extremely disturbing, making it difficult to cope with the day-to-day tasks of living, let alone the challenge of deciding whether to file a formal complaint. Acknowledging and dealing with these reactions directly, perhaps through one or more of the modalities mentioned in this book (such as a self-help group, individual or group psychotherapy), will minimize the interference of these reactions in your attempts to arrive at a decision that is right for you. In fact, such reactions may be the source of valuable information for you, may be helpful to you in reaching a decision.

EDUCATE YOURSELF ABOUT LAWS, PRINCIPLES, STANDARDS

Educate yourself regarding the laws, ethical principles, and professional standards regarding therapist-patient sex. The professions have asserted forceful prohibitions against any therapist engaging in sexual intimacies with a patient. It is not unlikely that you were unaware of such prohibitions at the time you were involved with your therapist. In Vinson's (1984) study, not one of the patients who had been sexually involved with a therapist had been aware of either the prohibitions or the complaint procedures. Furthermore, your therapist may have attempted to indoctrinate you with a number of false beliefs about the legitimacy and "healing power" of sexual involvement with him or her.

Other therapists, attorneys, and consultants may help you in this process of education. Yet, in our experience, the learning can be enhanced if you can, perhaps with the help of these resource people, obtain copies of the relevant documents, such as ethics codes, procedures for filing complaints with the licensing board, and so on. These documents can be obtained by writing to the central office of the professional association or to the relevant state licensing board. When you have your own copies of the documents, you can review the information first hand. You will be less reliant on second-hand information and the statements of "experts."

This process of self-education can produce a number of positive side effects. It may enhance your sense of self-esteem and confidence. It may make you feel more "in control." It may help make your decisions represent truly informed consent. It may widen your sense of options; you'll likely become aware of new possibilities.

CONTACT OTHERS

See if you can contact anyone else who has been through a similar experience. You can learn from them as well as feel empathy and support from someone who has "been there." This will likely help you to feel less alone and isolated, less stranded in a horrible situation. If you do not at present know anyone else who had made it known that he or she was sexually intimate with a therapist, consider contacting one of the self-help or advocacy organizations listed in Chapter 6. (At some point you may even consider starting your own self-help group or patients' rights organization.)

In addition to talking with others who have been in a situation similar to yours, consider reading the published accounts of those who have been sexually exploited by their therapist. *Betrayal* (Freeman and Roy 1976) is a vivid account of how a woman became sexually involved with her therapist and later successfully sued him. The description of the trial is fascinating.

The civil case, *Roy* v. *Hartogs,* was a landmark in this area. Unfortunately the book is out of print, but many public libraries as well as second-hand book stores have copies. *Therapist* (Plaisil 1985) is another first-person account of a woman's involvement with her therapist and later malpractice suit against him. Be aware that popular movies such as *Still of the Night* and *Lovesick* constitute highly unrealistic fictional accounts of such involvement, and embody many destructive myths. They are comparable to *Uncle Tom's Cabin* and *Birth of a Nation* in the harmful and completely false stereotypes they present.

CONTACT MENTAL HEALTH PROFESSIONALS

Consider contacting mental health professionals who are knowledgeable in this area and using them as consultants. As mentioned earlier, they can support you in your learning. Have they had any experience with the complaint process? Can they identify other practitioners who might serve as valuable consultants? Are they aware of court decisions or licensing board actions that are just being made public? Do they know of any research-in-progress or just-published literature in this area? In summary, what information, questions, or advice do they have that might be helpful to you?

Be aware of any biases that seem to be influencing an individual therapist whom you contact. Some therapists, for example, may be quite uninformed about this area. Some may be so outraged at the conduct of your previous therapist that they devote great energy to attempts to convince you that you should file complaints immediately with the court, with the licensing board, and with the ethics committee. Others may be so concerned about the horrible public image (let alone high malpractice premiums) that this phenomenon creates for therapists that they will act vigorously to influence you not to file. Still others seem to identify so closely with their fellow professionals (and to view all patient complaints as fictitious or a manifestation of unresolved transference issues) that they will attempt to discount what you have to say, to treat it as illusory, a fantasy, or at least trivial and of no real consequence. Such therapists may also attempt to blame you for instances of sexual intimacy. Recognize that a blaming or discounting attitude on the part of a therapist-consultant can have extremely harmful effects on your recovery. The more professional consultants you can speak with, the more you can become aware of such biases and take them into account when evaluating each consultant's information and advice.

You may also want to consider contacting a range of attorneys to gather additional information and consultation. Attorneys as a group are no more free of individual biases than are mental health professionals as a group, nor are they any less prone to take sexual advantage of someone whom they perceive as vulnerable.

Be aware that the mental health and legal professionals whom you contact for consultation and information may or may not be disposed to offer you "free" consultation. Some may respond to you on a human level and be willing to give you whatever input they can through a phone call or two or perhaps an office visit, all without charge. Others may provide some consultation at no charge because they feel a commitment to the profession. This responsibility to provide services pro bono (a Latin phrase meaning "for the good") is a part of many formal ethical frameworks. The Ethical Principles of Psychologists (American Psychological Association 1981), for example, states: "They contribute a portion of their services to work for which they receive little or no financial return." Other professionals, of course, may talk to you only if you begin paying their full fee. The "meter" is turned on immediately. Be aware of this range of approaches and make sure you clarify the ground rules before you entail a financial obligation.

Also be aware that even if you are only seeking some information and consultation, some professionals—both therapists and attorneys—may use this contact with you to try to influence you to become their client. The therapist may try to initiate weekly sessions of psychotherapy; the attorney may seek to represent you. In either case, make your wishes known to the professional and avoid responding to such insensitive pressure.

MAINTAIN RECORDS

Keep a diary and maintain records. Consider trying to write down, based on your memory and any records you might have (such as checkbook stubs of fee payments, letters, and such) of your involvement with your previous therapist. What led you to seek therapy? How did you find that particular therapist? What happened during and between sessions? What has happened to you since you've terminated? If you do decide to file a complaint, you'll need to reconstruct the sequence of events as part of the complaint process. Even if you decline to file charges, this systematic review of your experience may be an important part of your healing process.

Take notes on all your consultations. Facts that seem vivid while you are discussing them with a sympathetic consultant may fade in memory as time passes. If you receive conflicting information from various consultants, your records will enable you to identify the confusion and to seek further clarification and verification.

You may also want to note your impressions of each consultant. If you later decide to reenter therapy, you can review what you have written about each mental health consultant to see if any of them might be a good candidate for your new therapist. Similarly, if you decide to retain an attorney to advise and represent you in the complaint process, you can review your impressions of any attorneys you've consulted to see if you're satisfied with one you've already dealt with or if you want to seek further.

CONTACT RELEVANT LICENSING ORGANIZATIONS

Once you've learned about the formal standards prohibiting a therapist's sexual intimacy with a patient, contact each of the organizations that investigates complaints. Be aware that there are great differences among these organizations: their structure, their nature, their jurisdiction, their authority, and the steps they can take.

One possibility is filing an ethics complaint with a professional association. Some of the major associations are listed in Chapter 2 along with the specific passage from their ethical codes that prohibit therapist-patient sex. In order for the ethics committee to investigate a complaint against your former therapist, the therapist must be a member of that organization. If you do not have convenient access to a professional directory (a public or university library may have these directories), you can call the organization (such as the American Psychiatric Association or the American Psychological Association), give the name of your therapist (without saying that you are considering filing a complaint), and ask if the therapist is a member.

Some therapists may be members of more than one professional organization. As an example, a given therapist may be a psychologist who specializes in psychoanalytic approaches to family therapy. She or he may be a member of the American Psychological Association, the state psychological association, the local (city or county) psychological association, the American Psychoanalytic Association, and the American Association for Marriage and Family Therapy. You may have to do some detective work (meaning making some inquires by phone) to see if you can find out to what professional organizations your previous therapist belongs. **Professional organizations, acting through their ethics committees, have no authority to revoke a therapist's license, to stop him or her from practicing, or to grant monetary rewards.** We emphasize this point because patients who have filed charges with professional organizations have so frequently told us that the organization did not make this fact sufficiently clear. In most cases, if the ethics committee finds the therapist to have violated ethical standards, it can take one or more of the following actions: (1) expel the therapist from the organization and notify the membership of the expulsion, (2) suspend the therapist for a given period of time, (3) formally censure or reprimand the therapist, (4) require the therapist to obtain formal supervision in his or her work, (5) require the therapist to undertake continuing education courses, and (6) require the therapist to enter personal therapy for a period of time.

Once you have identified the professional associations to which your previous therapist belongs, a good strategy is to call each association and ask its ethics committee to send you all available information regarding their complaint procedures. Once you've read their literature carefully, you're ready to call them to ask any questions you might have. Such questions (if they are not answered clearly in the literature they mailed to you) might include:

- What is the average time it takes for a complaint to be resolved? (This will give you an idea of how long the process is likely to take.)
- On what evidence will the committee make its judgment? For instance, can you appear before the committee in person? Will your former therapist be required, invited, or allowed to make a personal appearance before the committee? If so, can you be present? If you can be present, will you be allowed to ask questions?
- Will your former therapist be allowed to see the materials you submit? (It is likely that the answer to this will be yes; the rationale is to enable the therapist to respond fully and specifically to the charges you make.) If so, will you be allowed to see the materials your therapist submits in defending him- or herself so that you can attempt to rebut specific assertions?
- Over the past several years, approximately how many therapist-patient sex complaints were filed, about what percentage were found in favor of the complainant or respondent, and what sorts of actions did the committee require of therapists found in violation of the prohibition against sexual intimacy? Ethics committees will safeguard the privacy and confidentiality of individual case deliberations, but should maintain general statistics—useful for a variety of purposes—on the types of complaints they receive and the dispositions (which do not reveal individual identifying information). If the committee has failed to keep any such statistics, does not participate in any such program evaluation and self-monitoring of their work, it may provide one index of the seriousness with which they take their task.
- Will you be notified in writing on the specific result of your complaint? Clarify exactly what sort of information, if any, you will be given. Some committees may answer affirmatively to this question, but years later you may receive a variation of the following form-letter: "We have investigated your complaint and taken appropriate action. Thank you for contacting us." Some people who file complaints may feel intensely betrayed to have taken the trouble and risk to "go public" by filing a formal complaint, to wait years for a resolution, and then to be met by a stonewalling response. Whether you will receive notification of the result of your complaint may or may not influence your decision to file, but having honest information that is not misleading about such notification is an essential part of your arriving at an informed decision about whether to file.

- What other notification, if any, will the committee make? For example, if the therapist is found to have violated ethical standards, will the committee notify its full membership? Will the committee notify the appropriate licensing board?

When making such a call to obtain information, be sure to note who is providing the information. At this stage of your consideration regarding whether to file a complaint, you may not feel ready to give up your privacy. It may be best to begin the conversation with the representative of the professional organization with some variation of the following statement: "My former therapist, who is a member of your organization, had a sexual relationship with me, and I'm trying to decide how I want to deal with it. If you could answer some questions about your complaint procedures, it would help me to decide whether to file a complaint. Because I'm not sure whether or not I'm going to file a complaint, I'd like to talk with you on an anonymous basis and not mention my therapist's name or my own name."

Although the organization will have no legitimate need to know your name to answer your general questions about the complaint procedures, if you decide to file a complaint, you will need to sign a formal complaint. There is virtually no ethics committee that will investigate an anonymous complaint of this type. (Some ethics committee may investigate certain types of complaints on the basis termed *sua sponte*. In such complaints, the basis of the complaint is already in the public record. Thus if a therapist were judged by a malpractice court to have engaged in therapist-patient sex, the finding would be a matter of public record. Anyone may then, on an anonymous basis, send the record of this judgment to an ethics committee, which may then decide to investigate.)

A second possibility for complaints is the state licensing board. As mentioned in Chapter 2, all states license psychiatrists and psychologists, over half license social workers, and a few license marriage and family counselors. The Department of Consumer Affairs or Department of Health Services or a similar branch of your state government will be able to tell you which licensing boards exist in your state and how you can contact them. By calling each board, you'll be able to find out which license(s) your former therapist holds. Be aware that your therapist may hold more than one license. For example, a physician who practices as a therapist may hold both a license to practice medicine and a license as a family therapist.

The procedures for gathering information from the licensing board(s) are similar to those for gathering information from professional organizations, and you may want to ask many of the same questions as were listed above.

When talking with representatives of either professional associations or licensing boards, ask yourself if the representatives seem competent and informed? Do they treat you with respect and courtesy, or do you feel like you're being brushed aside, that you're a bother? Do they return your phone calls promptly? Do they give clear, specific, and informative answers to your questions? These initial contacts are your initial and first-hand indication of how you and your complaint are likely to be treated by this institution.

If you receive unsatisfactory responses to your questions (for instance, the person on the phone is rude to you, or gives you misinformation), you may want to follow up on it at some later point in your life (after you have made and implemented your decisions regarding filing a complaint). You may want to bring it to the attention of the president of the organization and the board of directors (if it is a professional organization), or to your elected representatives and appointed office holders (if it is a state licensing board). If this step does not produce a satisfactory response (for example, if your letter is ignored), you may conclude that such organizations respond best to public concern. Such concerns can be generated and expressed through your local mental health agency, through letters to the editor of the local paper, through special writings (for instance, longer pieces in the New York *Times* or in the *Newsweek* "My Turn" column), and so on. One of the self-help and advocacy groups listed in Chapter 7 may offer you valuable information, ideas, and support in bringing your concerns to public attention.

The third possibility for complaints is a malpractice or other tort suit. The descriptions in *Betrayal* or *Therapist* may give you some idea of what such trials involve, but an attorney is in a position to provide the most sound information. You may have to shop for an attorney whom you genuinely trust and can work with (*Therapist* gives an agonizing account of some of the frustrations in seeking an adequate attorney). If you know someone who has filed such a suit, he or she may be able to tell you the names of attorneys who will be good possibilities (as well as the names of attorneys to avoid). Be assertive in asking the attorney about his or her training and experience. How many cases has he or she tried? Has the attorney handled cases specifically in the area of therapist-patient sex or more generally in the area of malpractice? Is the attorney enthusiastic about taking the case? Do you get a sense that the person will be committed to your case and will make every effort to represent your rights? Make certain it is someone whom you feel good about; you will be working with that person over a long course of time on a very important matter.

Clarify what your working arrangement will be. Will you be paying the attorney a retainer or will he or she be paid a percentage of the judgment (assuming the court decides in your favor), or both? Once you've described your complaint, what is the attorney's evaluation? Does it seem like a strong case or an uphill struggle, a long-shot? What are the possible outcomes?

Will the attorney return your calls and be available to answer your questions in the years ahead? Will the attorney want to work closely with you, explaining the strategies and inviting your input, or will he or she expect you to be passive? Be sure to make your expectations known and find out if you (and your case) and your attorney are well matched.

MAKE YOUR OWN DECISION

After you have completed this process of gathering information and advice, you will know—as well as you can at this point—what the possibilities are and what they entail in terms of time, commitment, work, and possible outcomes. The question now becomes deeply personal. What is in your best interests? What do you really want to do? Clarify your own motives. What do you want to achieve, to strive for? In light of your current situation, your distress, your values, your wants and needs, what choice seems best? Filing no complaint (at least at present)? Pressing your complaint through one of the channels? Through more than one channel (either simultaneously or sequentially)?

If you decide not to pursue a complaint at present, but feel you might want to file sometime in the future, find out what the "statute of limitations" is for each procedure (civil suit, licensing board, and ethics committee). Be aware of any time limits on your decision.

RETAIN AN ATTORNEY

If you arrive at a decision to file a complaint, seriously consider retaining an attorney (though of course you may have consulted attorneys on an informal basis previously to gather information). An attorney who is retained by you can help you implement your decision in the manner that best ensures your legal interests. For instance, if you decide to file a complaint with an ethics committee and also a civil suit, the attorney can advise you how filing both simultaneously or filing them sequentially can affect the outcome of each. It may be advantageous for you to file your complaints in a particular order. (Filing complaints also influences when, and under what circumstances, your previous therapist learns that an investigation will be undertaken. This may have considerable implications. For example, licensing boards, upon receiving a complaint, may first send an undercover investigator to the therapist. If a sexual intimacy complaint has been filed by a female patient, the investigator may be a woman presenting herself to your former therapist as a patient. If the therapist attempts to seduce her, your case is obviously strengthened. However, if you have simultaneously filed a civil suit and an ethics complaint, and your former therapist has been notified, then he or she is likely to be on "best behavior" at least until the complaint is resolved.)

* * *

For almost every complainant with whom we have talked, the complaint process has been long, arduous, and frequently frustrating. For most of them, however, their decision to pursue a formal complaint was, in retrospect, one about which they feel good and which was an important part of their recovery.

10

Guidelines for Lawyers Working with Patients

Consumers look to the courts for protection against and requitement after victimization by mental health professionals. The states, charged with guarding the welfare of consumers, have used their licensing function and administrative law systems to prevent and contain such victimization. Whether in criminal, tort, or administrative law actions, in cases of exploitation of patients by psychotherapists, the judicial systems have been viewed as deterrent, arbiter, rehabilitator, and vindicator. Endowed with this multiplicity of roles, the systems have struggled to be responsive to the varying needs of those involved in such disputes.

Attorneys handling cases of sexual intimacy between psychotherapists and their patients are dealing with problems specific to these types of cases, which frequently differ markedly from other instances of malpractice. Because of this difference, many patients who live in areas of the nation that are not adequately served by attorneys who have handled such cases have been told that they do not have a cause of action, and have been denied a day in court. Increasing attention by media to such cases has increased the awareness of many consumers, and there are increased demands for referrals to attorneys in various parts of the country to undertake such cases.

This chapter is addressed to such attorneys in particular. Just as some subsequent therapists have unwittingly caused iatrogenic damage to patients who have been sexually involved with previous therapists, so also do some attorneys. Sought out by this population to represent them and vindicate them, attorneys frequently find themselves faced by clients who do not trust them, who are demanding, who alternate between passivity and stubborn refusals, and who generally are seen as "difficult" clients. In response, many attorneys either refuse to take such cases or, having accepted the responsibility, unwittingly damage their clients.

SOME COMMON SCENARIOS

The following three vignettes are fictional. Yet they represent experiences commonly faced by many patients who seek legal representation.

Example 1: A distraught client calls attorney A, with a rambling story of having been sexually used by a therapist for a period of years. Attorney A responds with a question as to whether the client was raped. When the client responds negatively, the attorney states that the client must have enjoyed the sexual involvement; why else did she return weekly over such a long period of time? The client cannot answer the question and the attorney states that the client does not have a cause of action.

Comment: This is by far the most frequent scenario whatever the gender of the attorney. Overlooked by the attorney is: (1) the power differential between patient and therapist, and (2) the strength of the transference. The patient looks to the therapist for help, and when the therapist states that sex is a part of therapy or that it is "good for" the patient, the patient is too powerless to protest or to question. Also, the transference may cause the patient to view the relationship with the therapist as a "lifeline" without which he or she cannot exist. If there is no other choice available, if the patient views the relationship as the only hope of survival, consent is not an issue. Frequently, the patient's vulnerability is exploited by the therapist. The trust demanded by the therapist as a *sine qua non* of therapy is betrayed. The patient then is severely damaged. Attorneys who have not represented clients in malpractice suits involving sex with therapists should: (a) refer them to a therapist who is knowledgeable about the problem unless the client is already in therapy; (b) ask for literature regarding the topic from their therapist; and (c) be aware that blaming the victim or attributing sexual motivation to the patient can be damaging.

Example 2: Attorney B listens sympathetically to the distraught client who tells him about being exploited by her psychotherapist. He tells her that he believes her, is interested in taking the case, and that she should bring in all her records. The client expresses anxiety about turning over the material, whereupon the attorney tells her that she must trust him. She has heard those words before, but feels that if she doesn't stay with this attorney, no one else will believe her and take her case (parallel to her feelings that if she refused the sexual advances of her therapist, he would not continue to see her). She brings the records. The attorney locks her in the office and forces her to perform fellatio on him. Feeling powerless she does as she is told.

Comment: Multiple victimization is not unusual in this type of case. Frequently these patients have a history of incest and/or child abuse, as well as rape and possible spousal abuse (see Chapter 4). The repetition of this exploitive behavior by psychotherapists and attorneys convinces these patients that there is no one in the world who can be trusted. These are the patients likely either to need hospitalization or to attempt suicide.

Example 3: Attorney C is consulted by a psychotherapist who is being sued by a woman for sexual involvement. The therapist explains that the woman was not a patient at the time; she had terminated therapy with her after she fell in love with her and did not begin a personal relationship with her until three months later. She explains that she had been careful to tell her that they could not see each other before they terminated therapy. The attorney agrees to take the case. She assumes that ending the therapy terminates the therapeutic relationship.

Comment: The literature shows that professional ethics committees, licensing boards, and triers of fact have not tended to be sympathetic to this argument (see Chapter 3). Expert witnesses are usually in agreement that there is no specific temporal criterion that allows termination for the purpose of beginning a sexual relationship. Concerns regarding premature cessation of therapy without dealing with the presenting problem, need on the part of the patients for further therapy in the future, and similarities of such relationships to incestuous involvements preclude acceptance of this therapist's rationale.

WORKING WITH SEXUALLY ABUSED CLIENTS

Clients who report having been sexually abused by a therapist require particular care. If their therapist was male they usually have lost trust in men. However, they are almost always ambivalent and may still have strong positive feelings about their previous therapist, so that negative statements about that therapist may bring out protective responses. They may not reveal necessary evidence, may be hesitant even to give the name of the therapist, and may test you to see if you can be trusted. Many feel guilty and responsible for what happened and will attempt to elicit a blaming response to you (see Chapter 8). Or they may attempt to test your response to their sexual advances in order to assess where your sympathies lie. They will expect disbelief and fear it. They will await mistreatment at your hands with resignation, for many have experienced victimization before and have come to accept it as an inevitable part of their lives.

DECIDING TO REPRESENT A CLIENT SEXUALLY ABUSED BY A THERAPIST

You consider yourself a fairly experienced, mature torts attorney. You are contacted by a potential client who claims to have been sexually involved with his or her therapist. Your secretary sets up an interview and you recall the well-publicized case in which $4.6 million was awarded to a patient who sued her former psychiatrist for malpractice as a result of sexual intimacy under the guise of therapy (*Walker* v. *Parzen* 1981).

What must you do to prepare yourself to meet and interview this potential client? What remedies can you offer to the potential client? What issues will you most likely confront in litigating your client's claim?

The following discussion is designed to be of help to attorneys representing clients who have been sexually intimate with a therapist. Because the various jurisdictions in which such a claim may arise have different statutes and case laws that govern the resolution of certain issues, the material will attempt only to identify potential issues rather than to set forth specific procedures.

ISSUES IN DEALING WITH CLIENTS WHO HAVE BEEN SEXUALLY ABUSED

Prior to your initial intake interview with your potential client, become familiar with the basic literature available in social science publications about the problem of sexual intimacy between therapists and their patients. There is a body of theoretical, clinical, and research literature that has accumulated in the last 15 years that addresses the problem and reveals the nature of therapist-patient sexual intimacy and its consequences (see Chapters 2-5).

It is important that you examine your own attitudes concerning such a client. Your attitude toward the client in the initial interview will determine the course of the attorney-client relationship. Recognition that these patients have been severely damaged in many instances will help you maintain the patience, empathy, and understanding necessary to assist such clients. As an attorney, you should not attempt to interpret motivation of the client or comment on causality of the incident. The ability to empathize and to offer support to these clients is of primary importance. If you feel that the responsibility for the sexual involvement rests with the client, you are at risk for further damaging the client. It is important to recognize that *the therapist is solely responsible for ensuring that sexual contact with the patient never, under any circumstances, occurs.* If the patient was seductive, desired sex, or in any way attempted to involve the therapist in activities that were not therapeutic, it was still the *sole responsibility* of the therapist to deal with that behavior and explore it professionally and therapeutically rather than to exploit it. To do otherwise was to act in an unethical and clinically destructive manner. *There is never an ethical or clinical justification for a therapist to participate in sex with a patient.* If this is not your position, it is strongly suggested that you refer your potential client to a different attorney.

Often a client will display uncertainty and will vacillate about proceeding with the case. Missed appointments, outbursts of anger, confusion, ambivalence about bringing in requested documentation—all are characteristic of these clients. They often will be angry with you but will not be able to express that anger directly. The oblique expression of hostility might underlie missed appointments, and gentle but firm direction is necessary to avoid such behavior. Since most of the clients are women and most of the therapists men, if you are a male attorney it is important to realize that the mistrust and anger you evoke may have little to do with you personally but are understandably misplaced feelings from the previous relationship with the therapist. Regardless of your gender, you, as an authority figure, are a target for the release of such feelings of being betrayed by another person, by an authority, by a professional. In order to understand the dynamics of this process more fully, you may wish to read Chapter 8.

INITIAL INTERVIEW

Your secretary ushers your potential client into your office and after the usual introductions and formalities you are ready for the actual interview. The establishment of rapport is the first task. Many of these clients need the opportunity to talk about what has happened to them and to hear that you understand the problem. They have often been hurt by family and friends who do not understand what has occurred or the depth of the distress and confusion they feel. Although you do not need detailed information of any depth in this first interview, it may be desirable to let the client speak freely. Probing is not desirable at this point. Once the client has provided enough general facts so that you are able to determine if there is a meritorious claim, the question you must ask yourself is whether you believe the client is telling the truth. The most frequent defense asserted in these cases is that the sexual contact never occurred. If you have doubts, it is important that you refer your client for psychological evaluation as early in the handling of the case as possible. If the client is already in treatment it will help you to speak with the treating therapist if your client is willing to provide consent for the release of information. Obviously the resolution of the question of the client's veracity will dictate whether or not you agree to represent the client.

One of the most difficult phenomena with which to deal is the client's ambivalence and resultant vacillation in pursuing the litigation. This uncertainty may be difficult for you to accept, since it often impedes the necessary actions to be taken. Although the client took the initial step of contacting you, he or she may subsequently develop anxieties, guilt, remorse, self-doubt, positive feelings for the offending therapist, fear of the previous therapist, or other feelings that impede progress in the case. The client ultimately must decide whether to sue and it is important that the decision be an informed one. As an attorney you must advise the client, albeit gently, of the emotional upheavals appurtenant to a lawsuit.

From a practical standpoint, your client must be sufficiently motivated to bring a lawsuit. A client who is poorly motivated at the beginning could walk away during the pendency of the suit. Also, there need be sufficient available damages and collectability to justify an attorney undertaking the case, be it on an hourly basis or a contingency. Recent decisions on the part of insurance companies to place caps of $25,000 and/or $250,000 have not as yet been tested in the courts, and settlements have continued in excess of such amounts.

Once you are satisfied that the truthful client wants to pursue the claim, that there are resources available to justify the case, and you have undertaken to represent the client, there are several other important steps:

1. Ensure that the patient is being treated by a competent therapist and/or participating in a support group (see Chapter 6).

2. Communicate with the therapist about the progress in therapy and the readiness of the patient to undertake the required activities such as depositions, and so forth.

3. Discuss with the therapist the client's plan to go on with life after the suit, pointing out the possibilities of the loss of the suit.

4. Share information with the therapist about the ambivalence, anger, or other symptoms displayed by your client that are bothering you. It is important that you understand the reasons for the behavior. Frequently attorneys reject clients because they appear to be "unmanageable" or "difficult," while all that is needed is reassurance or limit setting, depending on the client and/or the circumstances.

5. Ensure that all discussions between you and the therapist are known and agreed to by your client. You may want to consider a three-way meeting attended by you, your client, and the client's therapist.

GOALS

What type of remedy is your client seeking? There are four possible courses of action that may be undertaken (as outlined in Chapter 2): filing a complaint with the national, state or local professional organizations of which the therapist is a member or with the state administrative licensing authority; criminal prosecution; or a civil action for damages against the therapist.

Ethics codes of all of the professions state specifically that sex between the therapist and a patient/client is unethical (see Chapter 2). These codes not only indicate that the therapist who engages in such behavior is committing an unethical act, but also that the conduct falls below the standards of care of that profession. The attorney has the obligation to develop evidence that the violation of an ethics standard was a proximate cause of the injury to the patient.

The therapist who is licensed by the state can have that license revoked through a report to the proper agency. A determination is made after a constitutionally guaranteed right of hearing and confrontation by the complaining witness. In representing your client, you may want to participate in the administrative proceedings, thereby providing additional support to your client as well as educating yourself as to further details of the claim. Through the administrative process you may be able to judge the demeanor of the defendant-therapist as well as evaluate the credibility of your client in a trial-like setting.

However, the process also assists the defense. There are an increasing number of attorneys who avoid participation either by the client or themselves in such proceedings since the accused therapist may utilize the proceedings to gather material and evidence to be used in defense of a later civil lawsuit. (Of course this works both ways.) This is especially true in cases where the administrative hearing is recorded and is later available. You should be aware that since an administrative hearing is considered somewhat similar to a criminal hearing the respondent therapist need not testify, so that the only testimony may be that of your client who can later be impeached if there are any discrepancies in the client's testimony.

The advantages an administrative procedure may provide your client include revocation of the therapist's license as well as allowing your client a practice run prior to civil litigation. In recent years the tendency in some states has been to look to suspension and probation rather than revocation, since a therapist can practice under a different license or designation after having been revoked and then is beyond the reach of the licensing board. (Several of the reported cases that deal with administrative hearings are: *Dresser* v. *Board of Medical Quality Assurance, Bernstein* v. *Board of Medical Examiners, Cooper* v. *California Board of Medical Examiners, Solloway* v. *Dept of Professional Regulation, Colorado State Board of Medical Examiners* v. *Weiler.*)

Generally, the standard against which the administrative procedure measures the therapists' behavior is provided by statute. (In California, for example, the Business and Professions Code provides the applicable statutes.) These statutes may aid the civil litigation by establishing the breach of the therapist's duty, should there be any doubt.

The results of administrative hearings are generally *not* admissable, unless based solely upon the admission of culpability of the therapist.

Prior to the early 1980s, the focus of actions involving therapists engaging in sexual relations with patients was either administrative hearings or criminal prosecutions. Criminal prosecutions of therapists engaging in sexual relations with patients is an old occurrence, but one that is now being considered again in several states (see below).

In the 1893 case of *Eberhart* v. *State,* a physician treated an epileptic girl of 13 by sleeping in the same room; eventually the doctor shared his patient's bed. The physician was convicted of statutory rape.

Another well-known case, *People* v. *Bernstein,* involved the criminal prosecution of a psychiatrist who engaged in sexual relations with his 16-year-old client. Dr. Bernstein was convicted of statutory rape.

Interestingly, both of these criminal cases involved charges of statutory rape, against which consent of the underage victim is no defense. More difficult is the clarification to the trier of fact when the victim is of age but not capable of consent because of vulnerability, the strength of the transference, and the significantly unequal power distribution. The expert witness becomes an essential part of the process at this point (see Chapter 11).

Recent efforts have been made to simplify criminal prosecution of therapist-patient sexual involvement by changing the statutes to state specifically that such activity on the part of the therapist is a felony or misdemeanor so that the question of consent is not an issue. Both Minnesota and Wisconsin have passed such laws but several attempts at new legislation in California have failed, in most instances foundering on the consent issue. Even with the addition of a rebuttable presumption clause it was not possible to obtain the legislation.

The 1970 American Law Reports Annotation Civil Liability of Doctor or Psychologist for Having Sexual Relationship with Patient, 33 A.L.R. 3d 1393 cites that "apart from *Nicholson* v. *Han* (1968) 12 Mich App. 35, 162 NW 2d 313, research has failed to disclose any case in which the courts have discussed or passed upon the civil liability of a physician or psychologist, as such, who while the client-patient relationship subsisted, had established a sexual relationship with a patient." In the last 10 to 15 years, more and more civil actions have been filed against therapists for sexual involvement with patients. Chapter 2 discusses the landmark decisions of *Zipkin* v. *Freeman* and *Roy* v. *Hartogs.* Despite the increase of such cases, the attorney seeking information about these cases may have difficulty because cases may settle and therefore do not become common knowledge, and even if such cases go to trial, the trial decisions are not reported in many jurisdictions. (One way to find them, however, is to contact services that compile data on cases in certain areas.)

A civil action against a therapist who has engaged in sexual relations with a patient will likely result in monetary compensation. Most civil actions are brought under the umbrella of professional negligence or malpractice. The primary difference between therapist malpractice cases involving sexual relations and those that don't is the issue of the standard of care. Whereas therapists' methodology of treatment may differ, the unanimous consensus of the professions is that therapists are not to engage in sexual relations with patients. Thus, the major issue of proof is that the sexual conduct took place (Schutz 1982).

ISSUES DURING PRETRIAL LITIGATION

Several alternative causes of action may be pled: professional negligence, assault and battery, breach of fiduciary duty, intentional infliction of emotional distress, fraud, undue influence, money had and received, willful misconduct, breach of contract, breach of implied-in-fact contract, and punitive damages.

Certainly the former patient is a proper plaintiff. Other potential plaintiffs may include the patient's spouse and/or children. However, the causes of action that a patient's spouse and/or children may make is much more limited.

If the patient and his or her spouse underwent therapy together—for example, marital counseling or family therapy—the spouse, even though he or she did not have sexual relations with the therapist, may be able to plead those causes of action predicated upon the therapist's professional negligence, that is, breach of fiduciary duty, breach of contract, breach of implied-in-fact contract, intentional infliction of emotional distress, fraud, and money had and received. Spouses who have jointly undertaken therapy with patients with whom therapists have had sexual relations have been successful in recovery against these therapists. Examples include:

Whitesell v. *Green.* The plaintiff and his wife underwent marital counseling with the defendant-therapist. Two weeks after the counseling concluded, the defendant-therapist had an affair with the former patient, wife of the plaintiff. The plaintiff sued for breach of the therapist's duty of responsibility. The defense was that the counseling relationship had terminated at the time of the affair. Jury awarded plaintiff $8,000 in general damages and $10,000 punitive damages.

Mazza v. *Huffaker.* Trial court instructed the jury that if it determined that the psychiatrist-defendant continued to treat the male patient after becoming sexually involved with the patient's wife, the jury could find malpractice. The North Carolina Court of Appeals affirmed the jury awarded damages of approximately $650,000, of which $500,000 was punitive damages.

Rosenstein v. *Barnes.* Plaintiff-psychiatrist brought action in Municipal Court against husband and wife for an unpaid bill of $5,400. When served with the complaint, wife informed husband that she had been having sexual relations with therapist for over ten years. (Initially husband and wife began treatment together for marital counseling.) During the trial the husband's case was settled for $20,000.

For those actions in which the spouse was not a patient of the therapist, other causes of action may be pled, for example, alienation of affections or loss of consortium.

Restatement of Torts 2d S683 authorizes alienation of affections actions: "one who purposefully alienates ones' spouses' affections from the other spouse is subject to liability for the harm thus caused by any of the other spouse's legally protected marital interests."

However, as noted in comment b of S683, several states have statutes ("anti-heart-balm statutes") that specifically forbid the bringing of an action for alienation of affections (California Civil Code S43.5, for example). The counter to anti-heart-balm statutes is an action for loss of consortium. By bringing an action for loss of consortium, however, the patient's past sexual conduct and subsequent change must be proved. This requires testimony by both patient and his or her spouse, which may result in damage to both and to the relationship.

The therapist who engaged in sexual relations with a patient is a proper defendant. Other potential defendants include the therapist's employer, the treating facility, whether hospital, clinic, or professional association of therapists.

STATUTE OF LIMITATIONS

One of the most frequently encountered issues in these cases is a statute of limitations concern, that time period within which a lawsuit must be commenced, and which is defined by statute in each jurisdiction.

A motion *in limine* (precluding the admissibility of certain evidence) should be made relative to the patient's past sexual conduct. Evidence Codes (for example, Federal Rule of Evidence 412 and California Rule of Evidence 1103) that limit the admissability of a victim's past sexual conduct in a criminal rape prosecution may provide authority.

Frequently patients are so damaged by their sexual involvement with the therapist that they are unable to face the truth about what has occurred to them. They may have strong ambivalence about the therapist. Often their feelings of guilt or complicity keep them from even considering filing a complaint or suit. Sometimes the therapist has told them that sexual contact is part of the therapy, or has blamed them for his or her loss of interest, and they feel so responsible for the damage they have suffered that they don't realize that the therapist has the responsibility. These patients do not know nor can they allow themselves to consider the possibility that the therapist's sexual conduct is malpractice.

The knowledge (which must be defined by the law of each jurisdiction) occurs, generally, when the patient consults with another therapist who advises the patient that such sexual conduct was not proper and therefore is the basis for an ethics complaint, a report to a licensing board, or possible malpractice claim.

Since different jurisdictions and statutes may be applicable to the various causes of action against the various types of defendant therapists, no specific time limit for these claims can be stated here. However, the attorney should be careful in evaluating the dates that may dictate when the statute of limitations begins to run: the date that therapy with the defendant commenced, the date(s) upon which the actual sexual conduct took place, the date upon which therapy with the defendant ceased, the date upon which therapy with the defendant may have resumed, whether or not the sexual relationship between the therapist and client continued after the therapist-patient relationship ceased and if so, the date this private relationship ended, the last date for which plaintiff was charged fees for professional services, and finally the date upon which the client discovered that the sexual conduct by the therapist was improper. (It should be noted here that the sometimes completely debilitating nature of the trauma resulting from sex with a therapist may preclude genuine or effective awareness for years.) It is also important to know how and by whom the relationship was terminated and under what circumstances, and specifically whether the patient was referred by the treating therapist to another therapist. Unless the statute of limitations has clearly run you should bring the action. It is also important to know that many professional association ethics committees and licensing boards have now abolished statutes of limitations in this type of action and decide each complaint on a case-by-case basis.

DEFENSES TO CIVIL ACTIONS

1. It never happened. The most common defense asserted in a case of this type is that the sexual contact alleged by the plaintiff never occurred. One reason for this defense is the refusal of the liability carrier to provide coverage if sexual activity is admitted.

Two related issues are: (a) whether or not the defendant's professional liability insurance covers sexual conduct performed under the guise of therapy, and (b) the importance of the plaintiff's attorney to develop corroborative evidence.

2. Statute of limitations. Both the plaintiff's and the defendant's attorneys must be aware of a possible statue of limitations issue. The defendant's counsel should test the claim early by way of a demurrer or

summary judgment, and if successful, avoid the costs and risks of further litigation.

3. Consent. As mentioned above, criminal prosecutions of therapists have brought convictions of statutory rape in cases of minors in which consent is no defense. However, for civil action, the issue of consent may be brought to bear.

The plaintiff's attorney should strongly urge that no "consent" can be given by the patient because of the professional relationship in which the therapist is always significantly more powerful. *It is the therapist's duty to avoid sexual contact.* The therapist is trained and the patient is entitled to rely upon the education and experience of the therapist. The consent issue may provide a defense to certain causes of action, for example, assault and battery. However, it should not be a defense to the causes of action predicated upon the therapist's duties to the patient.

4. Contributory negligence. The defendant-therapist may attempt to assert that the plaintiff-patient was contributorily negligent, that is, initiated the sexual contact. It is not unusual in states where such defenses are effective to have a jury assess a portion of the responsibility to the patient: the therapist was responsible for 80 percent of what occurred and the patient 20 percent. Just as with the affirmative defense of consent, it is the authors' opinions that this defense is not viable to the causes of action predicated upon the therapist's sole responsibility and duty to the patient.

5. Developing corroborative evidence. Unless the plaintiff is fortunate enough to discover a witness who can testify that sexual contact actually took place between the therapist and patient, as in *Rosenstein* v. *Barnes,* supra, in which a witness for the plaintiff testified that the therapist, the patient, and she all engaged in sexual relations together, the resolution of this issue will revolve around the credibility of plaintiff and the defendant.

In order to substantiate the plaintiff's allegations, any and all evidence that corroborates his or her claim must be developed. Such evidence may include:

a) any physical evidence—for example, patient described therapist's genitalia and/or scars in areas usually not expected to be visible to a patient who has not had sexual contact with the therapist.

b) similar modus operandis with other patients about which the complainant may know. Once the case becomes public (reported in the papers), other patients, some of whom may not have been in treatment at the same time as the plaintiff, may come forward to testify or to file their own suits.

c) writings emanating from the therapist, and/or

d) telephone bills displaying frequency of calls between patient and therapist (obviously this item alone is not significant evidence).

Much of this evidence must be developed after the therapist has completed a deposition. After such deposition the defendant's statement of facts should be tested. For example, the therapist testified that air conditioning ducts would have transmitted sounds of "lovemaking" to other parts of the building. Testimony of building manager revealed that ducts are baffled to abolish sound.)

VALUE OF THE CASE

During the pendency of the case, it will become necessary to sit down with your client to attempt to achieve agreement on the "bottom line" value of the case. Similar cases tried in your jurisdiction can help provide a measure of the conscience of the community in which the case is to be tried. Judges are generally not good authority on values of such cases since they are in all likelihood not accustomed to dealing with psychological injury. You may wish to study verdict and settlement reports contained within the Association of American Trial Lawyers monthly *Law Journal,* not limiting your study to sexual abuse in therapy but also any and all other purely psychological trauma cases.

The most important yardstick is the testimony that the attorney has available from a competent researcher as to the damage created by therapist-patient sexual involvement (see Chapter 11 on Expert Testimony). There are data available to show that such damage has far-reaching effects and can cause severe trauma (see Chapter 5).

Other important variables in your case will be the credibility of your client and expert testimony as to how this client, in particular, was damaged. The current treating therapist will be the key expert witness in this testimony.

"Special" damages are those that have been suffered by the victim and constitute out-of-pocket expenses necessitated by the therapist's conduct. This of course would include the cost of the original psychotherapy that damaged the client and the subsequent therapy needed to help the client recover from the trauma. The treating therapist will be able only to approximate what such treatment could cost, since many factors enter into the rapidity of improvement in therapy. The defense attorney will generally respond to the request for reimbursement for prior therapy with the claim that those sessions are not attributable to the conduct of the defendant since the patient originally sought therapeutic intervention for previous problems. The response is that the offending therapist not only did not help the underlying problem but compounded those problems far beyond their prior existence.

Another factor in evaluating prospective damages is the amount of insurance available that covers the defendant and the collectability of the defendant. In *Rosenstein* v. *Barnes* the jury returned a verdict in the total sum of $250,000, of which $125,000 was compensatory damages and the remainder for fraud. The defendant's insurance company was not, under the terms of its policy, obligated to respond to the fraud damages. However, in order to avoid further litigation and appeals the case was settled in the full amount of $200,000, with the insurance company paying that amount.

TRIAL

Perhaps the most important factor in the trying of this kind of case is the jury voir dire. The jury must be selected on the basis of attitudes and sympathies. If you practice in a state or judicial system where the judge undertakes the voir dire, you will not be able to ascertain those sensitivities. Factors such as personally having been in therapy or having had a family member in therapy should be considered. Willingness to award damages for psychological injury is also important to assess. During voir dire it is important that therapeutic issues be raised in order to assess awareness and sensitivity to such issues.

It is important that the client be carefully prepared but not rehearsed. The shock of hearing diagnosis, prognosis, and description of sexual activity in open court can so distress the client that the trial will have to be interrupted. Although one can never completely mitigate the impact, prior explanation of the necessity for exploring such issues can prepare the client for what is to follow. Rehearsal, on the other hand, can result in encapsulation and withdrawal so that the desired spontaneity will not be present. The balance is achieved through experience in working with this population.

When you interrogate your client, questions should bring out the history of the relationship with the defendant therapist, the reason for the original consultation, the way sexual intimacy began, and the way the relationship ended.

Cross-examination of the defendant therapist, if he or she takes the stand, should be done firmly but with respect. Interrogation should be probing to attempt to elicit the true nature of the relationship. General attitudes regarding the ethicality of sexual involvement with patients should be questioned. If the therapist claims that the therapeutic relationship was already over before the sexual relationship began, it is important to ascertain what steps were taken to deal with the transference (for example, was referral made to another therapist? Did the defending therapist seek consultation? What provision was made for the patient to have a therapist available if there were recurrent problems?).

The expert witness(es) should be knowledgeable about the research on the topic and/or have had clinical experience with this type of patient, because of the uniqueness of this patient population. It is important that the expert is able to testify that the events occurred as was told by the patient, that the conduct of the therapist fell below the standard of care, that as a result damage ensued, and what type of damage that was.

Closing argument should be direct and should eschew emotion except where the defense attorney allows "openings" that in turn allow you to respond emotionally in your rebuttal.

Finally, always remember that your assistance to this patient is a critical factor in allowing him or her to obtain redress and to move on with a life that has been seriously impaired.

11

Therapist-Patient Sexual Intimacy on Trial: Mental Health Professionals as Expert Witnesses

The purpose of this chapter is to present material that will help mental health professionals understand and function effectively in the legal systems. When expert witnesses are unprepared to discharge their duties, it is a tragedy for all concerned. Neither truth nor justice is served. The litigants—both plaintiff and defendant—are deprived of illuminating testimony regarding issues that can have a major effect on their lives. The jurors fail to receive the assistance they need in understanding matters that require specialized expertise. Even the expert witness is affected. As Sadoff (1975, p. 51) writes:

> There is nothing more pitiful than to see a leading member of the community, a distinguished physician, brought to his knees under cross examination because he is ill prepared and not in touch with current psychiatric principles. There are many legal tricks that the cross-examining attorney uses and the expert should be aware of these "tricks" and how to handle them.

The following issues should receive careful attention by all mental health professionals serving as expert witnesses.

THE FUNDAMENTAL TASK

The expert witness appears in the midst of adversarial proceedings but is not in an adversarial role. At most it can be said that the expert witness serves as an advocate for his or her expert opinion. He or she is not an advocate for the plaintiff, defendant, or any third party.

The fundamental task is to help the jury in their role as triers of fact. The expert witness is not in court to decide the case or to tell the jury how to decide the case. The task is educative in nature. The expert witness appears in court to bring to the jurors' attention certain inferences that are based on scientific or professional knowledge and expertise not possessed by the jury.

This is a difficult shift in perspective for many mental health professionals. They may be accustomed to attending to their patients' rights and interests, and to serving as advocates for them. Furthermore, when they work with attorneys, the attorneys virtually radiate an advocacy stance. The discussions are so often peppered with phrases such as "winning," "prevailing over the other side," "helping our side," and "gaining a victory." This is appropriate for the attorney, who plays an adversarial role. But the mental health professional must be aware of the ways in which such bias undermines and corrupts the integrity and effectiveness of the expert witness.

The expert witness is not a hired gun, selling his or her "opinion" to the highest bidder. Nor can testimony ethically be created or "shaped" in order to enrich a plaintiff, exonerate a defendant, or advance a purely personal point of view. The expert witness has a responsibility to fulfill the functions required by the court, and must resist all enticements—explicit or subtle, monetary, emotional, interpersonal, or ego-enhancing—to compromise this charge.

A section of Chapter 7 was devoted to exploration of the personal biases, conflicts, and countertransference that could interfere with the therapist's ability to render effective treatment to those patients who have been sexually intimate with previous therapists. Such factors must also be honestly and scrupulously examined by professionals preparing to serve as expert witnesses.

It is important to stress here that avoiding bias and the temptation to present a distorted picture to help one side win does *not* mean that the expert witness has no opinions. For example, a psychiatrist called by one of the attorneys may have conducted extensive assessments of both the plaintiff-patient and the defendant-therapist and may have concluded that the patient indeed suffered massive damage as a result of sexual intimacy with the therapist (or, on the other hand, that no intimacy occurred and that the charges are due to other factors). This opinion does not constitute "bias" as we are using the term, and the expert does no more than fulfill his or her task by serving as an advocate of this opinion in court. The responsibility is twofold. First, the opinion must be based on a professional assessment (rather than, say, a conviction that either all patient-plaintiffs or all defendant-therapists are always telling the truth, or the fact that an attorney paid the expert $1,000 to manufacture bogus opinions that would help win the case). Second, the expert must be honest—that is to say, must tell the truth, the whole truth, and nothing but the truth—in presenting this opinion in court.

THE ADVERSARIAL PROCESS

The expert witnesses enters an arena of fierce adversarial struggles. "We no longer have the simpler methods of trial by ordeal and trial by combat; we have in their stead trial by advocacy" (Greenspan 1978, p. 137). From this at times brutal, sly, manipulative, technicality-bound contest, truth and justice are presumed to emerge.

Thus the witness must attempt to fulfill the educative function in the midst of trained legal professionals who use every method the law allows to win. Because the attorney who originally calls the expert witness to the stand obviously thinks the testimony will be helpful, that attorney will be inclined to present the witness in the best possible light. He or she will want the witness to appear prestigious, knowledgeable, well-trained, experienced, competent, objective, and profoundly wise. The witness can expect help in presenting a clear explanation of his or her professional opinions, the factors that led to the formation of those opinions, and the relevance of the opinions for the case at hand. Of course the attorney will want to emphasize those aspects that will tend to win the case for his or her side and will want to ignore, discount, or deemphasize aspects that may hurt. The expert witness is dependent, to a large degree but not completely, upon the nature of the questions asked.

During cross-examination, the expert witness will encounter the strategy that the other attorney thinks will minimize the damage or perhaps even be favorable to his or her side. The choice of strategies ranges from politely leading the expert to reconsider opinions based on new information to making the expert look like a fraud, a scoundrel, or a fool. Under such circumstances, one often feels attacked and experiences an urge to respond defensively. Rarely do the defensive maneuvers accomplish much beyond eroding the witness's credibility.

Keeping clearly in mind the fact that one must maintain a nonadversarial stance within an extremely adversarial process is crucial to the effective functioning of the expert witness.

QUALIFICATIONS TO SERVE AS AN EXPERT WITNESS

Holding a clear view of the fundamental task of the expert witness and the nature of judicial systems, mental health professionals are in a position to evaluate attorneys' requests that they participate as experts in the legal process. During the initial phone contact, we must make a preliminary judgment—subject to revision once you learn about the case in more detail—about whether we possess authentic expertise in the subjects at issue. Sometimes this is a hard judgment to make if the attorney is appealing to our ego and we don't want to shut the door on a possible source of income. The most honest and rigorous self-scrutiny is essential.

In *Jenkins* v. *U.S.*, Judge Bazelon, in writing the majority opinion for the U.S. Court of Appeals, quoted McCormick in an attempt to specify the criteria for serving as an expert witness.

> An observer is qualified to testify because he has firsthand knowledge which the jury does not have of the situation or transaction at issue. The expert has something different to contribute. This is a power to draw inferences from the facts which a jury would not be competent to draw. To warrant the use of expert testimony, then, two elements are required. First, the subject of the inference must be so distinctively related to some science, profession, business or occupation as to be beyond the ken of the average layman, and second, the witness must have such skill, knowledge or experience in that field or calling as to make it appear that his opinion or inference will probably aid the trier in his search for truth. The knowledge may in some fields be derived from reading alone, in some from practice alone, or as is more commonly the case, from both [McCormick, Evidence 13 (1954), citing authorities].

Judge Bazelon himself concludes: "The principle to be distilled from the cases is plain: if experiences or training enables a proffered expert witness to form an opinion which would aid the jury, in the absence of some countervailing consideration, his testimony will be received."

AVOIDING CONFLICTS OF INTEREST

If we conclude that we do in fact possess the requisite training and experience to serve as an expert witness in the case as outlined by the attorney in the initial phone conversation, the second consideration is: Do we have a current or former relationship with any of the parties in the case that would constitute a conflict of interest, that would bias our opinion? Thus if we play tennis every Saturday with the defendant or are business partners with the parents of the plaintiff, we would likely need to acknowledge that our testimony would either be biased or appear biased.

In certain cases, however, we may have a current or former professional relationship with one of the litigants, and the attorney may be asking us to offer the court our professional opinions about that relationship. For example, we may be the subsequent treating therapist for a patient who is suing a previous therapist. Because patients who initiate a legal action that puts their own mental or emotional state at issue effectively waive privilege, it is crucially important—as we stressed in Chapter 6—for all therapists who provide assessment and/or therapeutic services to patients who have been sexually intimate with previous therapists to ensure that those patients understand fully the limits of privacy, confidentiality, and privilege. Patients need to understand this concept fully at the beginning of assessment or therapy, as part of their legal and ethical right to informed consent to services. The therapist must always be aware that a patient's knowledge that whatever is said is subject to being repeated in the courtroom can disturb the therapeutic relationship. It is also true that no matter how often the patient is reminded of this lack of confidentiality, there is always the shock of hearing the therapist reveal a diagnosis, a prognosis, and deeply personal information in a public setting, the nature of which is adversarial.

WORKING ARRANGEMENTS WITH THE ATTORNEY

If the preliminary information leads you to believe that you would qualify as an expert and that you would not be creating a conflict of interest, the next step is to discuss with the attorney your needs and expectations regarding any potential working relationship.

Different mental health professionals have different work habits and requirements, so there is no comprehensive set of rules applicable to all. However, the fee arrangements should be clearly specified. What are your charges? Many mental health professionals find it best to charge neither a lump sum for a particular case nor specific charges for itemized services but rather for their time. This allows greater flexibility and also helps to establish that the professional is not being paid to produce a particular opinion. A favorite story of attorneys and expert witnesses concerns an attorney whose case had been severely damaged by the effective presentation of an expert witness called by the other side. When the attorney began to cross examine the witness, having little hope of poking holes in the logic of the opinion, he sought to imply that the expert was a "hired gun," had come up with the opinion in exchange for the fee.

"How much are you getting paid to state the opinion we've just heard?" asked the lawyer.

"I'm not paid for the opinion; I'm paid for my time," replied the witness.

"And just how much will you be paid for that?" sneered the attorney.

The witness replied, "That depends on how long you keep me up here."

All significant issues regarding payment need to be addressed. Do you expect to be paid in advance? Note that lawyers often require a retainer up front, before they begin work. Technically, are you being retained by the lawyer or by the lawyer's client (to whom do you submit your bills)? Will you be charging for travel time? Will you be charging for the time—perhaps days or weeks—you may spend in court waiting to be called to testify? Will you be reimbursed for expenses, or will you be expected to absorb expenses out of your regular fee?

Does the attorney clearly understand that if you are retained, for example, to conduct a psychological and neuropsychological assessment of the plaintiff, that your results will not be influenced by the fact that you are being hired by either the plaintiff attorney or the defense attorney, and that your results may not be helpful to—and may in fact be detrimental to—the attorney's case?

Address issues of work schedules, availability, and deadlines. When is the case scheduled for trial? When will the attorney need your data? Unfortunately, an attorney may place an initial call to you on Tuesday afternoon and say that he or she needs you to testify Thursday morning. The attorney brings all persuasive techniques to bear on you, failing to mention that the case has been scheduled for trial for several months and the attorney is just now getting around to some aspects of preparation. Be realistic in such cases. If you do not have adequate time to conduct a thorough assessment and to prepare an adequate presentation, it is unethical to take the assignment.

Can you expect the attorney to return your calls with reasonable promptness and to schedule meetings as needed? The demands that other trials may make on an attorney's life need to be realistically evaluated. Different attorneys have different styles for handling their work and availability. What is important is that you know the attorney's availability between the initial phone contact and the trial and that you judge that the availability is adequate for your needs. On the other hand, you need to let the attorney know of your availability and scheduling. Can you return calls with reasonable promptness and does your professional schedule allow you to schedule necessary meetings? Are you strictly a nine-to-five person, or do you work nights and weekends?

Will the attorney secure and supply to you, with reasonable promptness, whatever records you believe you will need to reach a professional opinion? If you are evaluating a patient-litigant, you may feel it necessary to obtain their school records, of hospitalizations and previous treatment records, military service record, and other documents that will serve as a baseline for and will inform your assessment. Note that if you do not review these documents, the opposing attorney will probably ask you in detail about your failure to do so.

Finally, you may want to ask the attorney what experience he or she has had trying cases in the specific area of therapist-patient sexual intimacy. Part of your task may be not only to educate the jury, once the trial begins, but also to educate the lawyer regarding this subject. Knowing the degree to which the lawyer has experience in this area will help you evaluate the nature and amount of education you will need to provide.

MEETING THE ATTORNEY IN PERSON

Once you have, through preliminary phone conversation, reached a tentative judgment that you would qualify as an expert witness in the particulars of the case, that you would not be creating a conflict of interest, and that you and the attorney can establish mutually agreeable working arrangements, ask for a face-to-face meeting. No matter how much can be clarified over the phone, there is no substitute for meeting in person.

Consider sending to the attorney, prior to the meeting, a letter summarizing the working arrangements agreed upon through phone discussion as well as any other important items. Thus if there was any misunderstanding, it can be cleared up. Furthermore, having a written copy of the working arrangements can prevent, or at least minimize, the creative tricks our memory can play on us regarding important decisions.

When sending the letter to the attorney, include: (1) your curriculum vitae, so that the attorney is familiar with your qualifications, especially those relevant for establishing your credibility as an expert witness; (2) research material you will be citing and other basic readings on therapist-patient sexual intimacy (how much and what type of material to include will depend in part on the nature of the case and in part on the prior experience of the attorney in trying such cases); and (3) a copy of the code of ethics and the standards for providers of services for your own discipline (and also for the discipline of the person being charged with sexual intimacy, if he or she is of a different discipline).

During the face-to-face meeting, briefly review the working arrangements and ask the attorney to present to you an overview of the case (including the nature of the charges and the adjudication system to be used, which will be discussed in the next section). What plan does the attorney have for both preparing for and conducting the trial? What role does he or she expect you to play? What other expert witnesses, if any, does the attorney expect to call? What expert witnesses will the opposing attorney likely present? Begin to map out a tentative schedule for trial preparation. During what time period will you be conducting an assessment, if required? During what time period will you be presenting your opinions to the attorney and preparing your testimony? Having the attorney lead you through your testimony on direct examination (more than once) is invaluable, as is having the attorney (or one of the attorney's law partners) subject you to anticipated cross-examination questions.

During the preparation phase, don't neglect your responsibility to educate the attorney regarding the strengths and limits of your expertise, the nature of the subject matter about which you'll be testifying, and all aspects of the professional opinions you'll be presenting in court.

THE METHOD OF ADJUDICATION

It is important for the expert witness to understand which of the legal systems will provide the hearing and will attempt to adjudicate the case. The two most likely forms are civil courts and administrative hearings.

Malpractice is a tort—a wrong done by one person to another. More specifically, it is injury to a patient due to a breach of the professional duties of skill or care or of their improper performance by a health care professional (Carpenter 1965). The professional fails to discharge adequately his or her professional responsibility: to possess and exercise such reasonable skill as is ordinarily possessed by others in the same line of practice. Adhering merely to local or regional standards of care is no longer held adequate in some states (*Naccarato* v. *Grob*). The criteria for determining adequate care are: (1) that the professional must possess learning, skill, and abilities that others in similar practice in the United States ordinarily possess; (2) that the professional must exercise the same kind of care and diligence in the application of this knowledge; and (3) that the professional must use reasonably good professional judgment in carrying out his or her duty (Feld 1971).

Torts may be divided into three types (Shapiro 1984, p. 136): An "intentional wrong" is a tort done purposefully, a "reckless wrong" is a tort resulting from a conscious disregard of a known risk; "negligence" is not deliberate but rather results from the failure to know something that should have been known. Obviously, negligence is easiest to prove.

To prevail in a malpractice action, a plaintiff-patient must demonstrate, through a preponderance of the evidence, that the injury was proximately caused through the practitioner's act or omission. "Injury" includes not only death, physical damage, and damage to mental health, but also emotional distress and loss of income. The establishment of malpractice generally requires the testimony of expert witnesses, as the issues are generally outside the knowledge of the jury (Carpenter 1965).

When malpractice actions are adjudicated in favor of the plaintiff, the court attempts to make the wronged person "whole" again, usually through a monetary award. In administrative hearings, on the other hand, no monetary awards are given. As discussed in Chapter 2, administrative hearings are attempts to adjudicate complaints filed with the state boards that license mental health professionals. In most cases, a professional who has been found guilty of engaging in sexual relations with a patient will have his or her license suspended or revoked.

Changes in the Business and Professions code of many states have simplified the administrative law process considerably. The statement that sexual relations between psychotherapist and patient is cause for loss of license would appear to eliminate the need for proving negligence, sexual abuse, quality of care below community standards, and other more nebulous concepts to allow concentration on the simple question: "Did this therapist engage in sexual relations with this patient?" Unfortunately, this is generally not the case.

The expert may still be asked to review the complaint(s) filed against a therapist in order to determine if the treatment the patient reports receiving meets the standard of care practiced by members of the professional community.

A clear understanding of the system—of its special rules and regulations—within which the complaint will be adjudicated is essential.

FORMING AN OPINION

As described earlier, there are different roles for the expert witness. The expert witness may be called to testify exclusively about the nature and meaning of research and theory in the area of therapist-patient sexual intimacy. This may require no examination of any of the litigants. The expert witness may be called to testify about a long-standing professional relationship with one of the litigants. For example, the witness may be the subsequent treating therapist of the plaintiff-patient. The expert witness may be called to testify about a psychiatric or psychological assessment of one of the litigants, performed at the behest of an attorney during preparation for the trial.

In forming a professional opinion, the fundamental task as described above must be kept in mind. The task is not to "win" for a particular side but to assist the trier of fact. But there is another responsibility that is of great importance: recognition that the work done as an expert witness will likely have great impact on the lives of those involved. This does *not* mean nor imply that one distorts or misrepresents opinions to "help" someone. What it does mean is that when interviewing the plaintiff, defendant, or anyone else as a procedure for forming a professional opinion, one recognizes, appreciates, and respects the fact that the person is a human being. Bias, disrespect, motivations to hurt and destroy, and so on, are as out of line, unethical, and unacceptable in this context as they would be in a therapeutic relationship.

One basis for this responsibility to work with others, particularly the plaintiff and defendant, in a humane way is the fundamental ethics. For example, the first line of the Ethical Principles of Psychologists (American

Psychological Association 1981) is, "Psychologists respect the dignity and worth of the individual and strive for the preservation and protection of fundamental human rights."

A second basis takes account of the extreme vulnerability of many individuals participating in such legal actions. Mental health professionals are often keenly aware of the vulnerabilities of those whom they interview. Patient-plaintiffs, for example, may be brutalized by interviewers who seek not to conduct a sensitive, comprehensive, and valid assessment for the defense but rather to obtain, say, highly personal information about sexual activities that are to be quoted out of context in the "assessment report" and the trial.

A third basis is practical: Many if not most assessment techniques are heavily dependent for their power and validity upon a genuine rapport between the interviewer/test-administrator and the person being assessed. The research has shown how sensitive many tests are to administrator variables. Clearly, a mental health professional who is out to destroy a patient-plaintiff is not only acting unethically and exploiting the patient's vulnerability but also establishing conditions under which valid assessment is all but impossible. No matter whether the mental health professional is retained by the plaintiff or defense, no matter whether he or she is assessing the plaintiff, defendant, or some third party, a good-faith professional effort—free of hidden agendas and predetermined results—cannot be replaced with either a "whitewash" or a "smear-job."

A fourth basis is the fundamental task: the responsibility to serve the court in the interests of truth and justice rather than fill an adversarial role fighting for one side or other, a theme to which we return repeatedly because of its central importance in this phase of our professional work. Sadoff (1975, p. 35) writes that

> once the expert takes the witness stand and begins testifying, his allegiance belongs to the court, in the interests of justice. This may sound like an unattainable ideal, particularly when viewed from a practical point of view, but the court and the jury will look to the expert witness as a neutral, scientific individual who is presenting opinion in the light of impartiality, despite the fact that he may be called by one side or the other."

This orientation must be maintained through every phase of serving as an expert witness.

COPING WITH NERVOUSNESS

Most mental health professionals experience understandable anxiety when asked or required to appear in court. It is a strange and unfamiliar setting, and adversarial procedures are aversive to many therapists. As the trial date approaches, the nervousness may become quite extreme.

A few commonsense methods may be helpful in making the experience less aversive.

First, prepare fully. For many of us, there is a feeling of security in the process of detailed preparation and in the resultant status of being as fully prepared as possible. Thus much of our anxiety becomes sublimated—and serves a good end—rather than becoming a distressing and disabling terror. The anxiety tends to remain at a level sufficient to motivate us but not so high that it overwhelms us.

Some of this preparation—such as double-checking the accuracy of our scoring of psychological and neuropsychological tests or making sure that our knowledge of the field is completely up-to-date—we can do on our own. Other aspects are best done with the attorney who will be calling us to the stand or with colleagues. As mentioned earlier, having the attorney rehearse our presentation and conduct a mock cross-examination is almost essential.

Second, talk to colleagues who have served as expert witnesses and read accounts of such trials. For example, reading *Betrayal* (Freeman and Roy 1976) and *Therapist* (Plaisil 1985) can give you a sense of how mental health professionals testified (both on direct examination and cross-examination) for both the plaintiff and the defense in sexual intimacy trials.

Third, find out where the case will be tried and visit the courtroom beforehand. This will serve several purposes. You won't have to endure the anxiety of getting lost on the way there, or not being able to find the building, or not knowing what floor the courtroom is on the day of the trial itself. You can become familiar with the courtroom, get a feel for its layout and accoustics. Thus you won't be in an unfamiliar setting when you actually arrive to testify. If you know what judge will be presiding over the trial, you might want to observe that judge in action, get a sense of his or her personality, demeanor, habits. The more familiar the situation is on the day(s) you testify, the less anxious you'll tend to feel.

APPEARING IN COURT

When you appear in court to testify, your attitude will affect your credibility with the judge and jurors. Being flippant, adopting a "know-it-all" stance, or failing to speak above a whisper are unlikely to make a positive impression on anyone. Most importantly, these and related tendencies will distract from the content of your professional opinion. Your attitude should reflect the seriousness of the issues being adjudicated. Similarly, your dress should convey respect for the court. An expert witness dressed in Bermuda shorts and a tank-top may feel "comfortable" but alienate everyone in the room.

Choose with care what you bring with you. The opposing attorney will almost inevitably have the right to inspect all materials you bring. In some cases they may even be entered into evidence. One of our colleagues, a psychologist serving as an expert witness, had all her testing materials entered into evidence. She had to leave the courtroom without expensive materials crucial to her professional practice.

TESTIFYING

The first principle—assuming of course that you are well prepared—is to listen carefully to each and every question. If you have reviewed your direct examination with the attorney countless times, you'll probably assume that you know exactly what he or she will be asking next. But the scenario may change for countless reasons, both intentional and accidental. Listen to the question, be absolutely sure that you understand it, then make certain that you know exactly what you want to say. If you don't understand a question, ask to hear it again or ask the attorney if he or she can phrase it in a different way. At some points, you may want to respond by saying something like, "I understand you to be asking . . . (phrase the question in your own words), and my answer is . . . ." A permanent record is being made of these crucial proceedings. Avoid careless or impulsive answers.

Shapiro (1984, pp. 81-82) provided an excellent example of a witness who listened carefully to a question (on cross-examination) and declined to get trapped in ambiguity.

Attorney: Now then, doctor, hasn't research shown that the MMPI is invalid?

Expert: I really cannot answer that question; would you be able to define what you mean by validity?

Attorney: Come now, you're a doctor, don't you know what validity is?

Expert: Certainly, counselor, but there is predictive validity, construct validity, and face validity—to name only a few. You have to define your terms more precisely before I can respond to the question.

Attorney: I withdraw the question.

All of us are human. You may realize that you've made a mistake; perhaps you've intended to say one thing and inadvertently said another. This realization may come immediately, or it may come while you are answering a subsequent question. If you become aware of such a mistake, ask if you may be permitted to correct it.

Second, acknowledge and respect the limits of your expertise. If you do not know the answer to a question, say so. Don't attempt to cloud the issue or to bluff your way through. The rigidity of the "know-it-all" not only tends to destroy credibility but also tends to be alienating. A little humility—especially if it is leavened with gentle and appropriate humor—is often very appealing. However, make certain that your humor is not "off key" in relationship to the seriousness of the proceedings.

Third, be absolutely honest. Your responsibility is to tell the truth and the whole truth. Yet expert witnesses may feel that some information should be withheld—even in the face of direct questioning—from the court. For example, some witnesses feel uneasy about having rehearsed the direct examination with the attorney. They are afraid that the jury will think that the testimony is fabricated, that the attorney told the expert exactly what conclusions to reach and what words to use. Attorneys attempting to cross-examine will often probe a witness for "secrets" and material about which the expert is uneasy. One attorney believed that he could elicit a lie from a witness whom he presumed would not want to reveal "rehearsed testimony" to the jury. He began his cross examination with a questions headed in that direction.

Attorney: During the lunch break, were you conversing with the attorney for the plaintiff?

Expert: (seemingly flustered and hesitant) Uh . . . well . . . yes, I did spend some time with her.

Attorney: Did you not in fact spend the entire hour in the conference room?

Expert: I guess it was close to an hour.

Attorney: Would you tell the court exactly what it was that you were discussing?

Expert: (long pause) I'd . . . uh . . . rather not.

Attorney: (addressing the judge) Will your honor please instruct the witness to answer the question?

Judge: The witness will answer the question.

Expert: Well, I'd rather not say this publicly, but the truth is, I was telling her that I didn't see how she could lose this case with such an unprincipled and sleazy attorney handling the case for the other side.

If you attempt to bend the facts—for example, to cover up your ignorance or to avoid evidence that would discredit the opinion you're trying to present—not only are you committing a serious crime but almost invariably you'll undermine your credibility and thus discredit your opinions and presentation.

Fourth, try to present your professional opinions and the facts and theories that led you to form them as clearly as possible. Remember that your task is to assist the jury. On the one hand, if you speak in abstract jargon, you may lose and alienate everyone, no matter how sound your ideas are. On the other hand, if you speak as if you were trying to explain a simple idea to a five year old, your condescending language and attitude will prevent clear communication. Wherever possible, use everyday language and give examples based on experiences or information that will be familiar to the jury. In a sense, you are serving as a teacher. Think about the teachers or lecturers who have been most effective in your experience—as well as those who have been boring, incomprehensible, and alienating—and see if you can improve your ability to communicate effectively.

Fifth, at some point you may become completely confused and not know what to do. The lawyer who originally called you to the stand will likely try to help you out, but this may be ineffective. At such a point, if all else fails, ask the judge for help. He or she is the authority in the court-room.

ADDITIONAL RESOURCES

Although we have tried to outline the major issues to which any potential expert witness should give careful and informed consideration, many readers will want to examine these issues in more detail and consult additional references. We recommend that all mental health professionals serving as expert witnesses become familiar with *Coping with Psychiatric and Psychological Testimony* (Ziskin 1984a), *The Psychologist as Expert Witness* (Blau 1984), *Forensic Psychiatry* (Sadoff 1975), and *Psychological Evaluation and Expert Testimony* (Shapiro 1984).

12

Preventing Therapist-Patient Sexual Involvement

At a recent American Psychological Association symposium (Bouhoutsos 1985c), discussant Nicholas Cummings, a past president of that organization, termed sexual intimacy between psychologists and their patients a "national disgrace." He called for firm and unequivocal measures to deal with this problem. Unfortunately, there has been little research to answer the question of what works to prevent therapists' sexual involvements with patients. Despite the millenium-long existence of this problem, it has been treated with benign and sometimes malicious neglect and there have been few suggestions for either remediation or prevention. Research on the topic has usually been done for dissertations, since funding has generally not been available from either governmental or private foundation sources (Sinnett and Linford 1982). A recent request for funding from the American Psychiatric Association to obtain empirical data on frequency of therapist-patient sexual involvement was denied. The study had to be funded independently. A petition to create a task force to study the problem of psychotherapist-patient sexual involvement with the focus on remediation or prevention was received with favor but not funded by the American Psychological Association. Because this is an area of discomfort for the professions (see Chapter 2) they appear to be resistant to taking the steps necessary for the creation of an effective program of prevention.

The trebling of malpractice insurance premiums for psychologists between 1984 and 1985 and the sharply escalating number of lawsuits being filed against members of all the mental health disciplines has brought the issue to the attention of practitioners and given impetus to the search for methods to prevent the problem. In reporting their findings, most researchers have agreed that changes are necessary in those systems charged with educating, controlling, disciplining, and licensing therapists. There is agreement, also, that there are no simple answers and that multiple changes in public policy as well as on an operational level are necessary if damage to patients from sexual involvement with therapists is to be prevented.

EDUCATION

The Professions

Rare is the training program for mental health professionals that selects students with any attention to their propensity for sexual involvement with patients. Is this omission due to our lack of sensitivity to the issue or to the difficulty in detecting characterological disorders at graduate school entry level? Perhaps it is for both reasons. There is a growing body of knowledge from therapists who have been supervising or treating these offending therapists (S. Smith 1981). Much more empirical research is needed in this area to determine if: (1) it would have been possible to identify these therapists when they were entering students and to exclude them from entry into the profession; (2) any of these therapists are amenable to conventional interventions such as psychotherapy or supervision; (3) any other interventions are possible; or (4) these therapists should be excluded from the mental health professions as soon as they can be identified.

Evidence has been cited that psychotherapists involved in sexually intimate relationships with patients tend to be older, well-established, and frequently prominent members of their profession (Butler 1975), who have graduated from excellent training programs. Lack of training does not appear to be a causal factor. There is also little indication that either exposure or nonexposure to current curriculum content covering sexual relations with or attraction to clients results in any significant difference in the frequency of involvement with clients (Gechtman and Bouhoutsos 1985). Variables that are not in evidence are the types of curriculum material to which these sexually involved therapists have been exposed, the method of presentation, and the effectiveness of both content and method. Research is necessary to assess these variables and also to investigate whether other information and/or methods of information transmission might have greater impact. For example, videotaped interviews with patients who have been damaged, discussions with therapists who have been sexually involved with clients, tapes of mediation sessions with both patients and therapists—all of these "in vivo" presentations might assist in making the information more immediate and meaningful. Whether exposure to such material would translate into behavioral change remains to be evaluated.

Mandatory inclusion of information about therapist-patient sexual attraction and involvement in training curricula of all mental health disciplines would at least guarantee that the issues would be discussed and understood. This requirement is important not only for its possible deterrent effect on those students who might eventually be at risk for sexual involvement with their patients, but also for the therapists who will encounter patients in their practice who have been sexually involved with previous therapists. Awareness of the scope of the problem and knowledge of methods to treat such patients are particularly necessary to avoid secondary traumatization by therapists not trained to work with such individuals.

In contrast to curriculum modification, which appears to be possible, a serious problem with little likelihood of direct intervention is that of modeling. The high frequency of sexual involvement of professors and supervisors with their students does not appear likely to be amenable to intervention in the near future. Even in those universities that have regulations forbidding faculty sexual involvement with students, the prohibition is usually limited to undergraduates. Yet graduate psychology students in particular appear to be vulnerable to such involvements and only later in their lives do they recognize the damage that has been done to them. There is also evidence that those same students tend to repeat such behavior when they are therapists (Pope, Levenson, and Schover 1979; Glaser and Thorpe 1986).

Agencies and Institutions

In addition to educating students in academic institutions regarding the exigencies of therapist-patient sexual involvement, attention should be given to agencies where they obtain their practical experience. The finding that 14 percent of therapist sexual involvement with patients occurs in agencies and/or institutions (Bouhoutsos et al. 1983) suggests the need for interventions at this level. A recent suit (*Birkner* v. *Michael Flowers and Salt Lake County*) involved a county named as codefendant with a therapist alleged to have engaged in sexual intimacies with a patient. It was determined by the court that a mental health professional employed by a county hospital, and sexually involved with a client, was known by the county facility's employer to have exhibited poor judgment in past job-related activities before the sexual involvement occurred. The suit included the county because of its alleged irresponsibility in not having taken steps to discipline or fire the therapist involved. In another recent case, where action was not taken against the employing institution, a therapist was found guilty of molesting eight women. He had been fired from an institution in another state over a similar offense. A letter in the current file from the therapist's previous supervisor detailed the reason for the firing; however, the therapist was hired and the eight women became his victims. This type of negligence is not unusual in overworked, underfunded bureaucracies.

One way to lessen the likelihood of such occurrences is to construct a staff selection and hiring procedure. A check sheet on each person interviewed should include information about the applicant's past positions, whether terminated or resigned and the reasons; whether the applicant had been involved in ethics, legal, or licensing actions and, if so, what were the charges and the result. There would also be space for notation of calls made to the licensing board of the state of prior employment plus any out-of-state licensing boards that might have taken action against the individual. Although this kind of screening appears to involve considerable paperwork, the computerization of records has simplified this task considerably. Unfortunately, many states and some of the professions are still in transition to more modern systems. It is also highly desirable to require telephone contact with prior employers. A history of sexual involvement with clients does not usually appear in letters of recommendation.

Within agencies and institutions, in-service training and evaluation, done on a continuing rather than sporadic basis, can also assist in avoiding therapist-patient sexual involvement. Sexual attraction to (or what is viewed as sexually provocative behavior by) patients can be stressful to a novice or to a distressed therapist (see Chapter 3). Consultation with other members of the staff who are nonjudgmental and knowledgeable about the issues might prevent the therapist from acting on impulse.

It is important for agencies and institutions to have clear and explicit written policies forbidding sexual involvement with clients, ex-clients, and clients' spouses/partners or significant others. Written evidence of this policy can also assist in the defense against suits of negligence. Written clarification of grey areas is also desirable, such as policies on dating of clients, dual relationships such as business ventures, and so on. Explicit statements regarding the unacceptability of sexual involvement with clients whether during the therapeutic hour or beyond, during the course of therapy or beyond, should be included. As pointed out in Chapter 3, it is not clear at the present time when the therapeutic relationship ends and what is necessary to terminate that relationship. Some researchers have used a three-month period after cessation of therapy as a time period to use for the purpose of examining incidence of sexual involvement between patients and therapists (Holroyd and Brodsky 1977; Bouhoutsos et al. 1983; Gechtman and Bouhoutsos 1985), but the choice of a three-month period does not in any way imply either positive or negative sanction to sexual relations between therapist and patient after such an interval. Attorneys have sought to use this arbitrary time period as a hiatus accepted by the professions after which therapists may begin a sexual involvement with patients. A recent survey (Gottlieb, Sell, and Schoenfeld 1985) has shown, however, that neither state ethics committees nor licensing boards have found psychologists not to be in violation if they have used the defense that the professional relationship had already been terminated prior to the onset of a social or romantic relationship, nor that such relationship had begun after any particular length of time. Futhermore, in June 1986, the American

Psychological Association Ethics Committee declared unethical all sexual intimacies with clients, even if the intimacies take place only after termination of the clinical services. Thus the presumption of the existence of a known time lapse before such sexual involvements are acceptable is in error.

Public Education

One of the most difficult problems in devising preventive educational strategies for the public is reaching and influencing the potential consumer of psychotherapeutic services. The primary difficulty is targeting the population at risk since we have not as yet been able to differentiate potential patients who would be at most risk for becoming sexually involved with a therapist. Added to the difficulty of identifying a target population is the reluctance of the mental health professions to warn potential consumers about the likelihood of damage. Many states have Consumers' Affairs departments and it has been suggested (Bouhoutsos 1983) that these agencies could require that written information be made available to consumers of psychotherapeutic services to explain what constitutes ethical practice. Another possibility would be to require a plaque in every waiting room similar to those used by Blue Cross to announce that the particular therapist is a Blue Cross provider, or those that encourage the patient to discuss finances if there are questions. The plaque would be a simple and inexpensive way to provide the information that sex is not a part of therapy, and that it is unethical and in some states illegal for any therapist to engage in sex with a patient. It is understandable that mental health professionals harbor fears that this warning might turn potential patients away from assistance that is really needed. Interestingly, patients who have been sexually involved with their therapists have taken a different, but also negative, position in discussing the usefulness of providing this type of educational information. Many maintain that no amount of warning would have deterred them from entering into a sexual relationship with their therapist because of their neediness at the time, their belief in the "specialness of the relationship," and their inability to refuse anything the therapist told them was to their benefit, including sexual relations.

Little research, if any, has been done to assess the effectiveness of the use of mass media in preventing victimization. In the last few years there have been a number of television programs and films dramatizing problems of incest ("Something about Amelia"), battered women ("The Burning Bed"), and sexual intimacy between patient and therapist (*Betrayal, Lovesick*). *Betrayal* (based on the Freeman and Roy book) showed the negative consequences of sexual involvement; *Lovesick*, a comedy, romanticized it. An assessment of benefit or harm to the audience of these two films would add to our knowledge of the usefulness of media in prevention. Other television programs have explored the issues in interviews with patients who were damaged and/or with clinicians who have expertise in working with these patients ("Hour Magazine," "Intimacy File," "Donahue Show," "Sixty Minutes," and so on). Print media such as popular books (*Therapist, Betrayal*) or magazine and newspaper articles have addressed the issue as have radio call-in psychology programs. Whether any of these mass media approaches have been successful in alerting the portion of the public that is at risk and thereby preventing these types of victimization is not known. Prevention research is beset with methodological problems and this topic has not been high on the list of research priorities.

Although large-scale empirical studies on the impact of media on the prevention of therapist-patient sexual involvement have not been undertaken, a recent dissertation (Vinson 1984) with an admittedly limited sample (n = 28) has shown that media coverage is on par with subsequent therapists as the source of information about complaint procedures. Additionally, the authors have received many letters in response to appearances on television or radio programs about therapist-patient sexual involvement. A few correspondents have asked for assistance in locating attorneys willing to undertake malpractice actions, or requested information about how to file ethics complaints. Some have detailed feelings of guilt and complicity in their own victimization and relief in discovering that others have experienced similar feelings. But most documented their first realization that they had been victimized. Frequently their responses were shock, outrage, and a desire to do something about the therapist who had victimized them. Many other issues surfaced, among them the need to confront the therapist in order to deal with the unresolved feelings; anger at the inability of therapists to recognize the harm resulting from their involvement with the patient; disillusionment with therapists as a whole; anger with the systems' problems that prevents reporting of those therapists who are exploiters; the need for continuing education courses for psychologists to emphasize the damage done to patients by their therapists who involve them in sexual activity; and, finally, the demand that something be done to stop the exploitation of patients.

CONTROL AND CONTAINMENT

Professional Organizations

Professional organizations have nominal responsibility for the problem of sexual intimacy between members and their patients. The phrasing of this statement makes explicit the basic problem: mental health professional organizations have no jurisdiction over nonmembers, who may practice without belonging to the associations. In contrast, state bar associations have total jurisdiction of their members; if an attorney is dropped from the bar association she or he cannot practice law. The American Medical Association at one time maintained control over almost all physicians through hospital privileges, which were generally granted only to members of their organization, the AMA. Since an antitrust action forbade making hospital staff membership contingent on AMA membership, the AMA has been in a similar position to other medical and mental health professional organizations—without the power to discipline practitioners who are not members and who resultantly are not bound by their codes of ethics. For example, only about one-third of the licensed psychologists in California belong to the California State Psychological Association. Therefore, if a nonmember becomes sexually involved with a patient, an ethics action by the state association is impossible, since the association has no jurisdiction over nonmembers.

If a psychotherapist belongs to a local, state, or national professional association, an ethics action by that organization is possible if a claim is filed. Procedure to be followed in a typical ethics complaint is demonstrated below.

Typical Ethics Complaint Procedure

1. Initial inquiry to central office; determination if member. If not, complainant told to check other levels of membership.

2. Form sent for completion and copy of ethical principles. Complainant asked to describe ethics principles that respondent violated.

3. Completed form received; investigatory subcommittee appointed; letter sent to complainant requesting further information and substantiating documentation and names of witnesses and copies of documentation if complaint appears to be valid. Complainant requested to waive confidentiality, and copy of complaint is sent to respondent.

4. Letter to respondent enclosing copy of complaint. Respondent requested to reply within 14 days with witnesses' names and documentation if complaint is to be contested.

5. Subcommittee considers evidence from both sides. Makes decision about recommendation to the entire ethics committee. Case is reviewed and recommendation made. Vote is taken on disposition of case, but subcommittee may not vote. If penalty such as expulsion handed down, submitted to board of directors of the organization for final disposition. Board may concur with ethics committee or make its own decision.

6. Complainant and respondent notified. Respondent may appeal on procedural grounds and formal hearing held.

But with which organization does one file? National, state, county, or local? How does the patient, who has been damaged and is therefore not' functioning optimally, negotiate the bureaucratic complexities of the various professional organizations to discover which has jurisdiction over the errant therapist? Even the determination as to whether the therapist with whom the patient was involved is a member of any of these organizations is a major undertaking. In fact, figuring out with whom to file a complaint is probably one of the major hurdles of the complaint process. Only 4 percent of cases of therapist-patient sexual involvement are reported (Bouhoutsos et al. 1983). Half of the patients in the California study did not know that such behavior was unethical on the part of the therapist. In a more recent study (Vinson 1984), 80 percent did not know they could file a complaint. Most patients do not know the differences among an ethics complaint, an administrative law action, a civil or criminal action, and they are certainly uninformed about the costs (in money, if any, and time, and emotional distress) or the advantages and disadvantages of each.

It is apparent that the unwieldiness of the systems is one of the elements responsible for the low rate of complaints. One positive step toward resolution of this difficulty would be an integrated complaint system, at least for ethics complaints. Wherever the complainant entered the professional organization system, the complaint should be forwarded to the level where the therapist holds membership. Ideally, the system should be interdisciplinary, since all of the psychotherapeutic professions are in agreement that they have a common problem that needs to be addressed, and injury to patients transcends disciplinary lines. Recent formation of interdisciplinary councils with joint legislative and funding purposes suggests that similar cooperative ethics efforts might be useful in dealing with the problem of therapist-patient sex. It is not at all unusual to have a mix of therapeutic disciplines in a single case, whether as previous therapist, treating therapist, expert witness for either defense or prosecution, or other related roles.

After patients have been educated about the necessity of filing an ethics complaint, have negotiated the complexities of determining whether their therapist is a member of a professional organization, and have ascertained which level of membership has jurisdiction over the complaint process, can the patient relax with the knowledge that justice will be served? This question is an important one since in many instances the primary reason given for reporting is containment—the concern that other patients not be damaged. However, the answer is not a simple yes or no. There are several problems involved, an important one being attitudinal. Members of ethics committees are volunteers who take time from their schedules to devote several years to review the actions of their peers in response to complaints filed with them by members of the public. Since ethics committee members are professionals and the complainant is a nonprofessional there is an implicit assumption of bias both on the part of the public and the profession itself. Some professionals have indeed articulated their view that the charge of ethics committees is the protection of the members of the association. The structure of the professional organization also lends itself to that purpose. For example, in most instances malpractice insurance is contracted with the parent professional organization and the loss of a suit is a loss to the profession, which in essence places the association in a conflict-of-interest position. The recent ruling by psychologists' insurance carriers to limit payments by a $25,000 cap in instances of sexual involvement, if adhered to, places the therapist beyond the financial reach of the client. In such instances a suit is generally not attractive to attorneys and the damaged patient is left without a "day in court." Most ethics committees attempt to maintain an arms'-length relationship with political and financial interests of the parent association, but attitudinally it is difficult to remain impartial.

In light of such potential problems and limitations, what can be done by the professions to assist in the prevention of their members' sexual involvement with clients? There are several steps that can be taken: (1) openly and candidly recognize the existence of the problem; (2) educate members about the unacceptability of such involvement and clarify the parameters of that unacceptability as outlined above (dual relationships, statute of limitations, duration of therapy, outside of office hours, and such); (3) provide ongoing information to members about the "at risk" practitioner, with information about ways to assess one's own vulnerability, awareness of sexual arousal by clients, ways to deal with that arousal, sensitivity to stress and burnout, and so on; (4) establish a distressed psychotherapist program with protection of confidentiality and a panel of well-trained consultants who have been made aware of their own potential bias; (5) support effective legislation to ensure permanent revocation of licenses of those who have been repeatedly sexually involved with patients; (6) require continuing education courses in ethics with special emphasis on dealing with sexual relations with clients and recognition of attraction to clients as a condition of license renewal; and (7) insist on the removal of CAPs (limitations or ceilings) for insurance companies' coverage of malpractice suits involving sexual intimacy.

Licensing Boards

Ultimate control of the practice of the psychotherapeutic professions rests with the agencies that issue and revoke the licenses under which they practice. This is a governmental function designed to protect the consumer, and such licensure of the professions has existed in the United States since 1639, when it began in Virginia. Psychiatrists are under the jurisdiction of the medical boards; psychologists in some states may be under the jurisdiction of the medical board or in other states may be under the jurisdiction of an allied health professions board with a potpourri of others such as chiropractors, podiatrists, and so on. The other mental health disciplines have only recently sought regulation and recognition through licensure. Social workers are now licensed in approximately 35 states; and marriage and family counselors are actively seeking licensure in a number of states. Boards charged with regulating these professions vary from state to state, although almost all have the same purpose and function: the response to consumer complaints, conducting hearings, and applying disciplinary measures (Bouhoutsos 1984). Most boards are plagued by several of the following similar problems.

The Unlicensed Therapist

In many states, although there are adequate licensing laws, local jurisdictions will not, or cannot for a variety of reasons, prosecute those individuals practicing without a license. Thus the state may go through the time-consuming, expensive process of revoking a license only to have the psychotherapist continue the rhythm of practice under another title without missing a beat. Frequently the titles "counselor," "therapist," "analyst," "minister," and "teacher" are not restricted and psychotherapists who have had licenses revoked can retitle their practice.

Inadequate Training

There are marked variations in requirements of education and clinical training that enable a candidate to sit for a licensing examination among the various disciplines and from state to state. The American Association of State Psychology Boards has been working on model legislation that, if adopted by all states, would be helpful in achieving uniformity in standards of acceptable training for admission to licensing exams. Equivalency provisions in licensing have been difficult to interpret and, despite preference among psychologists for professional schools in university settings (Bouhoutsos et al. 1985), there has been a proliferation of free-standing schools of psychology, which has made the establishment of adequate standards of professional training very difficult to achieve. Among the states, certification of schools is frequently under the jurisdiction of the Department of Education and often only minimal funding and physical plant are required to qualify. Usually there are no set curriculum requirements. Thus curricula vary and there is little possibility of requiring uniform course content on sexual intimacy between therapist and patient. This is a problem unique to psychology, with its genesis in academia and its continued scientific research emphasis; psychiatry and social work, which have control over preparatory programs and separation of the professional from the academic probably can move more quickly to require such course content.

Delicensure

In the late 1970s the trend toward consumerism and the move away from licensure resulted in "sunsetting" in some states. The reasons advanced for this decontrol of the professions was the desirability of competition and the possibility of allowing the marketplace to be run by supply and demand. The results made it immediately apparent that licensure is a necessary and basic safeguard for the consumer, despite the accompanying realizations that although such licensure is a potential safeguard in many areas, in actuality it is not very effective in cases of sexual intimacy between psychotherapists and patients. Why? The following two problem areas exemplify some of the difficulties.

Examinations

States have the obligation to screen applicants for licensure to determine if they have undergone the required education and training necessary to be admitted to the examination. There are national boards and examinations in psychiatry and psychology. For psychologists, the states decide which score is sufficient to pass the examination. Some states have chosen to allow reciprocal licensure from other states. The twofold examination that requires credential review plus written/oral examinations provides sieves to eliminate those individuals not sufficiently prepared educationally or professionally for the practice of the discipline. The written examination usually tests for theoretical and practical knowledge of the profession. Orals are used to gauge ethical awareness and knowledge of the laws under which the candidate will be practicing. Unfortunately, tests for ethical insensitivity still have not been devised and personality testing is not a prerequisite for licensure. Cognitive awareness of what constitutes ethical behavior frequently does not guarantee conformity to the ethics of the professions.

Monitoring

The most reliable predictor for future behavior is still past performance. Therefore, adequate and readily accessible records are a necessity. It is important to screen licensure applicants for convictions in other states on charges of sexual involvements with patients and to catalog all complaints on individuals so that therapists can be delicensed if they are recidivistic. Another preventive step would be to monitor those therapists who have had their licenses revoked or suspended. In one instance when a therapist's license was suspended, she told her patients that she had run into bureaucratic red tape, and she would now be seeing them for "vocational counseling." All of the patients signed statements that they agreed to this arrangement and she continued her practice exactly as it was before. Obviously, monitoring is necessary to preclude practice under another designation. Some of the other problematic aspects of monitoring are the lack of funds available in the states for the monitoring function, and the dangers inherent in maintaining surveillance on any group of individuals. Traditionally licensing fees have been low and it is possible to raise revenue by taxing the profession itself for its errant members. Perhaps such fiscal impingement would alert practitioners to the behavior that caused the additional taxation, and would be an effective modifier of the amused tolerance with which many in the professions have viewed the sexual transgressions with patients by their colleagues. Increased reporting in print of those members of professional associations who have been "defrocked" probably would have a similar effect. The tradition of nonnotification of the professions (and even of the complainants) has done a disservice to primary prevention of therapist-patient sexual involvement.

THE ADMINISTRATIVE LAW PROCESS

When the patient finally finds the agency with which to file a complaint, the proper forms have been completed, and the complaint has been determined to be meritorious, what are the remaining systems problems to be addressed? Although the process differs in states and boards and professions, the general steps are the same. A sample state process is described below.

Typical Licensing Complaint Procedure

1. Patient (or relative, therapist) telephones board and requests to file complaint. Complainant is sent typed form to complete and return. Form requests identifying information, dates, descriptive information, name of perpetrator, and so on. (If form is not returned, no case is filed; no record is kept.)

2. Completed form received by board; acknowledged.

3. Board staff determines jurisdiction and appropriateness. (If another agency, forwarded; if no jurisdiction, case closed.)

4. If appropriate, forwarded to investigations or to attorney general's office for assignment, depending on state.

5. Preliminary investigation reported on to board; charges dropped and case closed; or attorney general's office recommends filing of formal complaint. Board decides whether to close the case with merit, dismiss, or file formal complaint.

6. Complaint formally filed; case now public record.

7. Deputy attorney general assigned to case; settlement stipulation may be considered. Proposed to Board. If Board rejects proposal, sets date for hearing.

8. Case heard before an Administrative Law Judge (no jury, no members of board present).

9. Decision of judge presented to Board. Board reviews hearing records, may accept or refuse decision; establishes disciplinary action to be taken. Some states do not allow more severe sentences than those handed down.

After the complaint has been filed, interviewing the complainant is usually the next step. Investigators in many states have had little experience in this area and while they frequently have had police training, they are in need of special education in the sensitivities and needs of this population. It is not unusual to have patients completely incapacitated and nonfunctional for weeks after an insensitive interview. In some states, training tapes provide information about the research findings on the subject of therapist-patient sexual involvement, and about ways in which investigators can be helpful and nontraumatic to the complainants. Such materials should be available to all states through the American Association of State Psychology Boards or organizations of other professional licensing boards.

Time lag is a universal problem in the administrative law process. Similar to other judicial proceedings, the complainant is put on hold and in most instances cannot continue with life until there is resolution of the case. In many instances the patient has left the home, has no support, is emotionally disabled, and cannot work. Frequently family relationships have been damaged and there is no familial support. The long process can be so destructive that despite the danger to the public that the therapist poses it is sometimes necessary for the subsequent therapist to counsel a fragile patient not to report, even if that patient is willing. In addition to the stress of the time lag, it is not unusual for the complainant not to be contacted during the entire pretrial period. The anxiety, anger, and fear during this time can be overwhelming and disabling. In those areas where support groups are available (see Chapter 6) it is possible to sustain some modicum of adjustment; however, in rural areas or in states where no such groups exist, it would be highly desirable for the state either to assist in the formation of such groups or to contract with agencies for the provision of local services to victims of their licentiates.

When the case is finally over it is possible in some states that the complainant is not advised of the decision, and that the first news of the outcome is obtained by reading a newspaper account. This type of neglect of the complainant's right to know appears to be particularly ill advised with this patient population.

DISCUSSION

There is little likelihood that the problem of therapist-patient sexual involvement will soon be resolved. This problem is iatrogenically created and is therefore the responsibility of the systems that train, license, and employ those psychotherapists who damage patients. Until there is recognition and admission of the existence of the problem change cannot occur. Defensiveness of the professions serves only to postpone needed planning. Questions have been raised in a number of areas: How can we help patients deal with therapists who seek to involve them sexually? How can we help therapists who are experiencing life difficulties look for assistance and avoid becoming still more distressed by inappropriate behavior? How can we identify therapists who will use their professional identity to exploit patients and stop them from degrading their profession? What can subsequent therapists do to ameliorate the damage caused by former sexually exploiting therapists? How can the various systems be more responsive to the needs of both therapists and patients? Patients continue to be harmed by our lack of action in these areas. Lives are destroyed. The trust that patients and society at large give to therapists should not suffer further betrayal. Continuing inaction is intolerable.

RECOMMENDATIONS

Our recommendations are presented in the outline that follows. They cover prevention and control for professionals, agencies, licensing boards, and the public.

Prevention

The Professions

1. Modify selection process for admission to training programs to include attention to issues of therapist-patient sex. (Though not addressing therapist-patient sex in particular, Sarason [1985] has provided an excellent analysis and set of recommendations regarding selection procedures.)

2. Provide educational material on sexual attraction and therapist-patient sex to all members of professional associations, including information concerning distressed therapist program availability. Include information about the effects of therapist-patient sexual involvement and how to handle sexual attraction to patients in all mental health training programs.

3. Enunciate strict prohibitions against professor or supervisor sexual involvement with students to avoid dual relationships, negative modeling, and other negative effects.

Agencies and Institutions

1. Institute staff processes with attention to past sexual involvements with patients.

2. Provide continuous in-service training and evaluation plus consultation specific to problems of staff-patient sexual involvement.

3. Distribute written policies forbidding sexual involvement with patients, ex-patients, and patients' spouses/partners or significant others.

4. Clarify policies regarding dual relationships.

Licensing Boards

1. Target gatekeepers in the community for special education and consultation regarding therapist-patient sexual involvement: in particular the police, attorneys, judges, consumer affairs staff, and patients' rights advocates.

2. Require a plaque in the office of every licentiate specifically stating that sexual involvement between therapist and patient is cause for delicensure and listing the phone number where a complaint may be filed.

3. Require copies of ethics codes to be available on display in the office of every licentiate.

4. Prepare, publicize, and distribute pamphlets about sexual intimacy between therapist and patient and its negative effects.

The Public

1. Request copies of ethics codes from professional organizations and written material from Consumer Affairs offices for information on therapist-patient sex and if none are available request that they be made available.

2. Request articles in your favorite publications by writing to the editor asking for information regarding therapist-patient sexual involvement.

Control and Containment

Professional Organizations

1. Develop methods for dealing more effectively with nonmembers sexually involved with patients; develop lines of communication with local law enforcement and educate them on the topic.

2. Simplify the ethics committee's complaint process.

3. Educate the public regarding the availability of ethics actions.

4. Clarify, institute, and publicize more adequate ethics rules and procedures that mandate timely response.

5. Institute program monitoring and evaluation to measure the effectiveness and efficiency of your ethics committee's adjudication of complaints.

Licensing Boards

1. Address the problem of the unlicensed practitioner; negotiate with local jurisdictions to undertake legal action.

2. Deal with complaints in a timely manner.

3. Monitor adherence to standards.

4. Emphasize ethicality dimension in oral examinations of candidates for licensure.

5. Share records and track therapists with revoked licenses so they cannot practice in another state if revoked.

6. Simplify the complaint process.

7. Screen and train staff to deal with patients experiencing posttraumatic stress disorder.

8. Keep the complainants informed of the process and advise them of the outcome.

9. Institute a serious system of program monitoring and evaluation of your work in this area.

Therapists' Checklist

Despite the many limitations of checklists, these items are offered to assist in self-evaluation. Examining this list from time to time—especially during periods of great stress or "burnout"—can help ensure that we handle appropriately any "risk factors" associated with therapist-patient sexual intimacy. If we do seem to be in a situation involving increased risk, awareness can be a crucial first step toward prevention. Reviewing the following issues may be helpful in evaluating our own vulnerabilities.

1. Becoming preoccupied with personal problems and devoting large portions of therapy session to discussing these problems with a patient.

2. Playing "know it all" with a patient: providing authoritative answers to all the patient's questions and becoming angry when challenged or caught in an error.

3. Telling the patient to engage in certain kinds of sexual behaviors, so that you can derive vicarious enjoyment and feel a sense of control over someone else's sexuality.

4. Instructing a patient to refrain from sexual relations or to discontinue certain relationships, based on your jealousy.

5. Dressing or talking in a seductive manner.

6. Telling a patient to dress or talk in a seductive manner.

7. Meeting your patient for drinks, dinner, or a "date."

8. Scheduling your patient's session (at night, as the last patient of the day, and so on) on the basis of your sexual attraction rather than on the basis of the patient's clinical needs.

9. Discussing sexual issues and material with the patient on the basis of your sexual interests rather than on the basis of the patient's clinical needs.

10. Finding yourself sexually attracted to or aroused by the patient without examining this response in light of the treatment dynamics and the appropriate handling of this response.

11. Isolating the patient (for example, not referring to a physician for screening medical problems, to a psychologist for psychological and neuropsychological testing, to a colleague for adjunctive treatment or a "second opinion") so that you become the patient's only lifeline and so that any improper activity between you and the patient will more likely go undetected by others.

12. Isolating yourself (not seeking out customary consultation, supervision, support, and so on, from colleagues regarding your work with a particular patient).

Appendix B
Patients' Checklist

Many patients who have become sexually involved with their therapist have noted that they "didn't really know what was happening," or that "it all happened so fast," or that they "thought this was the way therapy was supposed to happen." The following checklist was created to help patients become aware of areas of possible risk or actual abuse.

This checklist, of course, is not comprehensive, and you may be concerned about attitudes, behaviors, or situations that are not on this list. A first step in resolving your concerns and avoiding therapist-patient sexual intimacy might be, if you believe it is feasible and advisable, bringing up your concerns with your therapist. Some therapists, however, may be so manipulative and intimidating that they preclude such questioning. If your therapist does not provide fully satisfactory answers to your questions or if you have concerns you are unable to bring up with your therapist, find one or more third parties who can help you understand what is going on and what course of action you wish to take. If you know other licensed therapists, you might ask them. You might contact the state agency that licenses therapists and put your questions to them. You might contact the state or national ethics committee and ask for consultation. You might want to contact one of the consumer self-help organizations listed in Chapter 6.

The major point is not to ignore or discount your feelings of being troubled or confused about what is going on. Don't assume that the therapist must be right, or that your doubts are only a function of the difficulties that led you to seek therapy. Don't try to sweep the danger signals under the rug or hope they go away if you don't pay them any attention.

1. Your therapist fails to explain treatment approaches and interventions in advance of implementation and does not obtain your informed consent for all procedures. If you begin asking questions or challenging the therapist's authority, he or she refuses to discuss the issues with you in a helpful way but rather attempts to manipulate you into unquestioning compliance. Some therapists may use anger, attempting to frighten you off from asking uncomfortable questions. Others may seek to make you feel guilty ("Here I am doing all these wonderful things to help you out of your desperate situation and you don't trust me!"). Still other may try to make you feel stupid ("I've had years of training—how could you hope to understand these complex ideas and treatments?"). You may meet a wall of questions ("What makes you want to know about this treatment at this time?").

168

And you may be threatened ("If you're going to waste my time and yours with all these irrelevant questions, why don't you just find another therapist right now!"). If your therapist does not treat you, your questions, and your legal right to informed consent with fundamental respect, you may be at risk for substantial damage from the relationship. One form the damage may take is a sexualized relationship.

2. Your therapist begins to devote large amounts of your therapy sessions to discussions of his or her own life, problems, and needs. An example of this focus on the therapist is provided by the scenario entitled "Role Trading" in Chapter 1. It is important to note that there is a legitimate therapeutic technique of "self-disclosure" in which the therapist may reveal something from his or her own experience in order to help the patient feel less alone in confronting a problem, to emphasize that the therapist is human, and to demonstrate ways in which the patient's problem might be faced. How does one tell the difference between appropriate self-disclosure and inappropriate self-centeredness? In appropriate self-disclosure, the disclosure will be prompted by an issue the patient has raised. The therapist's discussion of his or her own life will not dominate the session. The focus will remain on the patient's problem.

3. Your therapist gives you illicit drugs—such as cocaine—during the session or recommends that you secure such drugs and begin using them. The scenario entitled "Drugs" in Chapter 1 gives an example of this approach.

4. Your therapist drinks or invites you to drink alcohol during a session.

5. Your therapist suggests you discontinue meetings at the therapy office and replace them (or supplement them) with more relaxed meetings at your home, his or her home, or a motel.

6. Your therapist invites you to dinner or other "dates." See the scenario entitled "Time Out" in Chapter 1 for an example.

7. Your therapist begins using romantic names—"lover," "dearest," "darling"—to address you.

8. Your therapist begins sending you notes or letters declaring love.

9. Your therapist refuses to acknowledge the legal, ethical, and clinically based prohibitions against therapist-patient sexual intimacy. He or she begins explaining that such behavior is actually legitimate and will be beneficial for your problems.

10. Your therapist begins attempting to run your life in regard to your sexual behavior. This may take the form of prohibiting you from having any sexual relationships (due to the therapist's jealousy and attempts to increase your isolation and dependency) or of "prescribing" certain sexual practices (so that the therapist has the vicarious thrill of controlling your sexuality and can indulge voyeuristic tendencies in asking you to recount these "homework assignments").

11. Your therapist engages in any physical contact that is unwanted by you. Some legitimate "body therapies" such as Reichian work, bioenergetic analysis, Rolfing, and dance therapy may involve considerable physical contact. Even the "talking therapies" may at rare times involve physical contact. For example, if a patient is severely depressed and recounting a traumatic incident, a therapist may reassuringly squeeze the patient's hand. However, the therapist has no right to engage in contact if it is unwanted by the patient. Patients may feel free to tell their therapist that, for instance, under no circumstances do they want to be touched by the therapist. Furthermore, therapists have a clear responsibility to see that such contact is done only in appropriate ways for well-defined clinical needs. The scenario entitled "Hold Me" in Chapter 1 describes a therapist who violates this responsibility.

12. Your therapist kisses you passionately on the lips.

13. Your therapist touches your genitals or asks (or commands) you to touch his or her genitals.

References/Bibliography

Abell, J. M., and Strong, P. N. 1983. "The Impaired Professional: A Preliminary Survey of Six Professions." Paper presented at the annual meeting of the American Psychological Association, Anaheim, California, August.

Abramowitz, S. I., and Abramowitz, C. V. 1976. "Sex Role Psychodynamics in Psychotherapy Supervision." *American Journal of Psychotherapy, 30,* pp. 583–592.

Abramowitz, S. I., Abramowitz, C. V., Roback, H. B., Corney, R. T., and McKee, W. 1976. "Sex-role Related Countertransference in Psychotherapy." *Archives of General Psychiatry, 33,* pp. 71–73.

Adelman, H. 1981. "Publicizing Pedophilia: Legal and Psychiatric Discourse." *International Journal of Law and Psychiatry, 4,* pp. 311–325.

American Association for Marriage and Family Therapy. 1982. "Ethical Principles for Family Therapists." Upland, California.

American Medical Association, Council on Mental Health. 1973. "The Sick Physician." *Journal of the American Medical Association, 223*(6), pp. 684–687.

American Psychiatric Association. 1985. "Principles of Medical Ethics with Annotations Especially Applicable to Psychiatry." Washington, D.C.

_____ . 1981. "Principles with Annotations." Washington, D.C.

_____ . 1980. *Diagnostic and Statistical Manual of Mental Disorders,* third edition (*DSM-III*). Washington, D.C.

_____ . 1979. "Opinions of the Ethics Committee on the Principles of Medical Ethics With Annotations Especially Applicable to Psychiatry." Washington, D.C.

American Psychoanalytic Association. 1983. "Principles of Ethics for Psychoanalysis and Provisions for Implementation of the Principles of Ethics for Psychoanalysis. New York.

American Psychological Association. 1981. Ethical Principles of Psychologists (revised edition). Washington, D.C.

_____ . 1977. Ethical Principles of Psychologists (revised edition). Washington, D.C.

"APA's Ethics Procedures Upheld As Fair in Federal Court." 1985. *Psychiatric News,* May 3.

Asher, J. 1976. "Confusion Reigns in APA Malpractice Plan." *American Psychological Association Monitor, 7,* pp. 1, 11.

Bardwick, J. 1971. *Psychology of Women.* New York: Harper and Row.

Barnhouse, R. T. 1978. "Sex between Patient and Therapist." *Journal of the American of Psychoanalysis, 6,* pp. 533–546.

Baum, O. E. 1969–70. "Countertransference." *Psychoanalytic Review, 56,* pp. 621–637.

Beck, A. T. 1970. "Role of Fantasies in Psychotherapy and Psychopathology." *Journal of Nervous and Mental Disease, 150,* pp. 3–17.

Belote, B. 1974. "Sexual Intimacy between Female Clients and Male Therapists: Masochistic Sabotage." Unpublished doctoral dissertation, California School of Professional Psychology, Berkeley.

Benedek, E. P. 1977. "Training the Female Resident to be a Psychiatrist." *American Journal of Psychiatry, 134,* pp. 1244–1248.

Berman, A., and Cohen-Sandler, R. 1983. "Suicide and Malpractice: Expert Testimony and the Standard of Care." *Professional Psychology: Research and Practice, 14,* pp. 6–19.

Berstein, A. 1974. "The Genital Psychoanalyst." *Psychoanalytic Review, 61,* pp. 257–267.

Bernstein v. Board of Medical Examiners, 204 Cal. App. 2d 378, 22 Cal. Rptr. 419, 1983.

Birkner v. Michael Flowers and Salk Lake County. Civil No. C-82-8509, 1983.

Blau, T. 1984. *The Psychologist as Expert Witness.* New York: John Wiley.

Blum, H. J. 1973. "The Concept of Eroticized Transference." *Journal of the American Psychoanalytic Association, 21,* pp. 61–76.

Boas, C. V. E. 1966. "Some Reflections on Sexual Relations between Physicians and Patients." *Journal of Sex Research, 2,* pp. 215–218.

Boss, M. 1963. *Psychoanalysis and Daseinsanalysis.* New York: Basic Books.

Bouhoutsos, J. 1985a. "Sexual Intimacy between Psychotherapists and Clients: Policy Implications for the Future." In *Women and Mental Health Policy,* edited by L. Walker, pp. 207–227. Beverly Hills: Sage.

———. 1985b. "Therapist-Client Sexual Involvement: A Challenge for Mental Health Professionals and Educators." *American Journal of Orthopsychiatry, 55,* pp. 177–182.

———. 1985c. (Chair) "Patient-Therapist Sex: Search for Solution to a Systems Problem." Symposium at the Annual Meeting of the American Psychological Association, Los Angeles, August.

———. 1984. "Sexual Intimacy Between Psychotherapists and Clients: Policy Implications for the Future." In *Women and Mental Health Policy,* edited by L. Walker, pp. 207–227. Beverly Hills, Calif.: Sage.

———. 1983. "Programs for Distressed Colleagues: California Model." Symposium presented at the annual meeting of the American Psychological Association, Anaheim, California, August.

Bouhoutsos, J., and Brodsky, A. 1985. "Mediation in Therapist-Client Sex: A Model." *Psychotherapy, 22,* pp. 189–193.

Bouhoutsos, J., Holroyd, J., Lerman, H., Forer, B., and Greenberg, M. 1983. "Sexual Intimacy between Psychotherapists and Patients." *Professional Psychology, 14,* pp. 185–196.

Bouhoutsos, J., Van Gorp, W., Krupp, G., and Shag, D. 1985. "The Professional School Controversy: Attitudes of APA Members." *The Clinical Psychologist, 38,* pp. 55–59.

Brenneman, D. 1978. "Eisner Sex Surrogate: Patient Tells of Relations." Santa Monica *Evening Outlook,* January 12, pp. 1, 7.

Brodsky, A. M. 1977. "Countertransference Issues and the Female Therapist: Sex and the Student Therapist." *Clinical Psychologist, 30,* pp. 12–14.

Broverman, I., Broverman, D., Clarkson, F., Rosenkrantz, P., and Vogel, S. 1970. "Sex-role Stereotypes and Clinical Judgments of Mental Health." *Journal of Consulting and Clinical Psychology, 34,* pp. 1–7.

Burgess, A. W. 1981. "Physician Sexual Misconduct and Patients' Responses." *American Journal of Psychiatry, 138,* pp. 1335–1342.

Butler, S. 1975. "Sexual Contact between Therapists and Patients," Unpublished doctoral dissertation, California School of Professional Psychology, Los Angeles.

Butler, S., and Zelen, S. 1977. "Sexual Intimacies between Psychotherapists and Their Patients." *Psychotherapy: Theory, Research, and Practice, 139,* pp. 143-144.

California Association of Marriage and Family Counselors. 1977. Ethics Code. San Diego.

Carpenter, B. K. 1965. "Annotation: Malpractice Liability with Respect to Diagnosis and Treatment of Mental Disease." *American Law Reports, 99,* p. 600.

Cautela, J. R., and McCullough, L. 1978. "Covert Conditioning: A Learning-Theory Perspective on Imagery." In *The Power of Human Imagination: New Methods in Psychotherapy,* edited by J. L. Singer and K. S. Pope, pp. 227-254. New York: Plenum.

Chesler, P. 1972. *Women and Madness.* New York: Avon Books.

Cohen, F., and Farrell, D. 1984. "Models of the Mind." In *Review of General Psychiatry,* edited by H. H. Goldman, pp. 23-36. Los Altos, Calif.: Lange Medical Publications.

Cohen, R. J., and DeBetz, B. 1977. "Responsive Supervision of the Psychiatric Resident and the Clinical Psychology Intern." *American Journal of Psychoanalysis, 30,* pp. 51-64.

Colorado State Board of Medical Examiners v. *Weiler,* 402 P.2d 606 Col. 1965.

Colt, G. H. 1983. "The Enigma of Suicide." *Harvard Magazine* September-October, pp. 46-66.

Cooper v. *Board of Medical Examiners,* 49 Cal. App. 3d 931, 123 Cal. Rptr. 563 1975.

Cummings, N. A., and Sobel, S. B. 1985. "Malpractice Insurance: Update on Sex Claims." *Psychotherapy, 22,* pp. 186-188.

Cutter, F. 1982. "The Distressed Psychologist: Opportunities for Intervention." Paper presented at the annual meeting of the California State Psychological Association, San Francisco, February.

D'Addario, L. 1977. "Sexual Relationship between Female Clients and Male Therapists." Unpublished doctoral dissertation, California School of Professional Psychology, San Diego.

Dahlberg, C. C. 1971. "Sexual Contact between Patient and Therapist." *Medical Aspects of Human Sexuality, 5,* pp. 34-56.

_____ . 1970. "Sexual Contact between Client and Therapist." *Contemporary Psychoanalysis,* Spring, pp. 107-124.

Davidson, V. 1977. "Psychiatry's Problem With No Name: Therapist-Patient Sex." *American Journal of Psychoanalysis, 37,* pp. 43-50.

Demac, D. 1975. "Masters Blasts Innumerable Patient Rapes." *Hospital Tribune, 9,* p. 1.

Dorland's Medical Dictionary, 25th Edition. 1974. Philadelphia: W. B. Saunders.

Dresser v. *Board of Medical Quality Assurance,* 130 Cal. App. 3d. 506, 181 Cal., Rptr. 797, 1982.

Durre, L. 1980. "Comparing Romantic and Therapeutic Relationships." In *On love and Loving: Psychological Perspectives on the Nature and Experience of Romantic Love,* edited by K. S. Pope, pp. 228-243. San Francisco: Jossey-Bass.

Eberhart v. *State,* 34 NE 637, 1893.

Edwards, D. J. A. 1981. "The Role of Touch in Interpersonal Relations: Implications for Psychotherapy." *South African Journal of Psychology, 11,* pp. 29–37.

Eigen, M. 1973. "The Call and the Lure." *Psychotherapy: Theory, Research and Practice, 10,* pp. 194–197.

Feld, B. 1971. "The Psychiatrist's Liability for Malpractice." *Psychiatric Opinion, 8,* p. 6.

Feldman-Summers, S., and Jones, G. 1984. "Psychological Impacts of Sexual Contact between Therapists or Other Health Care Professionals and Their Clients." *Journal of Consulting and Clinical Psychology, 52,* pp. 1054–1061.

Fine, R. 1965. "Erotic Feelings in the Psychotherapeutic Relationship." *Psychoanalytic Review, 52,* pp. 30–37.

Finney, J. C. 1975. "Therapist and Patient After Hours." *American Journal of Psychotherapy, 52,* pp. 30–37.

Flescher, J. 1953. "On Different Types of Countertransference." *International Journal of Group Psychotherapy, 3,* pp. 357–372.

Forer, B. R. 1984. Personal Communication, November 8.

―――― . 1981. "Sources of Distortion in the Therapeutic Relationship." Paper presented at the annual meeting of the American Psychological Association, Los Angeles, August.

―――― . 1980. "The Therapeutic Relationship: 1968." Paper presented at the annual meeting of the California State Psychological Association, Pasadena, February.

―――― . 1969. "The Taboo against Touching in Psychotherapy." *Psychotherapy: Theory, Research and Practice, 6,* pp. 229–231.

Franklyn, T. 1978. "Sexual Transgressions against Patients." *California State Psychologist,* June, pp. 7–8.

Freeman, L., and Roy, J. 1976. *Betrayal.* New York: Stein and Day.

Freud, S. 1983. "Further Recommendations in the Technique of Psychoanalysis: Observations on Transference-love." In *Freud: Therapy and Technique,* edited by P. Rieff, pp. 167–180. New York: Collier Books. Original work published 1915.

―――― . 1953. "Three Essays on the Theory of Sexuality." In *Standard Edition of the Complete Psychological Works of Sigmund Freud,* volume 7, pp. 125–245. London: Hogarth Press.

Gaines, B. 1972. "Sex on the Couch: Analysts and their Patients." *Cosmopolitan,* September, pp. 152–155; 166.

Gareffa, D. N., and Neff, S. A. 1975. "Management of Clients' Seductive Behavior." *Smith College Studies of Social Work, 44,* pp. 110–124.

Gartrell, N., Herman, J., Olarte, S., Feldstein, M., and Localio, R. 1986. "Psychiatrist-Patient Sexual Contact: Results of a National Survey. I. Prevalence." Paper presented at the annual meeting of the American Psychiatric Association, May.

Gechtman, L., and Bouhoutsos, J. 1985. "Sexual Intimacy between Social Workers and Clients." Paper presented at the annual meeting of the Society for Clinical Social Workers. Universal City, California, October.

Geller, J. D. 1978. "The Body, Expressive Movement, and Physical Contact in Psychotherapy." In *The Power of Human Imagination: New Methods in Psychotherapy,* edited by J. L. Singer and K. S. Pope, pp. 347–378. New York: Plenum.

Geller, J. D., Cooley, R. S., and Hartley, D. 1981–82. "Images of the Psychotherapist: A Theoretical and Methodological Perspective." *Imagination, Cognition, and Personality: Consciousness in Theory*Research*Clinical Practice, 3,* pp. 123–146.

George, J. C. 1985. "Psychotherapist-Patient Sex: A Proposal for a Mandatory Reporting Law." *Pacific Law Journal, 16,* pp. 431–459.

Glaser, R. D., and Thorpe, J. S. 1986. "Unethical Intimacy: A Survey of Sexual Contact and Advances Between Psychology Educators and Female Graduate Students." *American Psychologist, 41,* 43–51.

Glauber, S. 1978. (Producer) "50 Minutes." Segment of the series "Sixty Minutes." New York: CBS Television, September 10 (originally shown February 19).

Glover, E. 1955. *The Technique of Psycho-analysis.* New York: International Universities Press.

Gottlieb, M., Sell, J., and Schoenfeld, L. 1985. "Social and Romantic Relationships with Former Clients: A National Survey." Paper presented at the annual meeting of the American Psychological Association, Los Angeles, August.

Greenacre, P. 1954. "The Childhood of the Artist: Libidinal Phase Development and Giftedness." In *The Psychoanalytic Study of the Child,* edited by R. Eissler, A. Freud, H. Hartmann, and M. Kris, pp. 47–72. New York: International Universities Press.

Greenbank, R. K. 1965. "Management of Sexualized Countertransference." *Journal of Sex Research. 1,* pp. 233–238.

Greenson, R. R. 1967. *The Technique and Practice of Psychoanalysis,* Vol. 1. New York: International Universities Press.

Greenspan, E. 1978. "The Role of the Psychiatrist in the Criminal Justice System." *Canadian Psychiatric Association Journal, 23,* pp. 137–142.

Gross, Z. 1977. "Erotic Contact as a Source of Emotional Learning in Psychotherapy." Paper presented at the annual meeting of the American Psychological Association, San Francisco, August.

Grossman, C. M. 1965. "Transference, Countertransference, and Being in Love." *Psychoanalytic Quarterly, 34,* pp. 249–256.

Grunebaum, H., Nadelson, C., and Macht, L. 1976. "Sexual Activity with the Patient: A District Branch Dilemma." Paper presented at the annual meeting of the American Psychiatric Association, Washington, D.C., May.

Hare-Mustin, R. T. 1974. "Ethical Considerations in the Use of Sexual Contact in Psychotherapy." *Psychotherapy: Theory, Research and Practice, 11,* pp. 308–310.

Harris, M. 1973. "Tort Liability of the Psychotherapist." *University of San Francisco Law Review,* Winter, pp. 405–436.

Hays, J. R. 1980. "Sexual Contact between Psychotherapist and Patient Remedies." *Psychological Reports, 47,* pp. 1247–1254.

Heimann, P. 1950. "On Countertransference." *International Journal of Psychoanalysis, 31,* pp. 81-84.

Holroyd, J. C. 1983. "Erotic Contact as an Instance of Sex-biased Therapy." In *The Handbook of Bias in Psychotherapy,* edited by J. Murray and P. R. Abramson, pp. 285-308. New York: Praeger.

Holroyd, J. C., and Bouhoutsos, J. 1985. "Sources of Bias in Reporting Effects of Sexual Contact with Patients." *Psychotherapy: Research and Practice, 16,* pp. 701-709.

Holroyd, J. C., and Brodsky, A. M. 1980. "Does Touching Patients Lead to Sexual Intercourse?" *Professional Psychology, 11,* pp. 807-811.

_____. 1977. "Psychologists' Attitudes and Practices Regarding Erotic and Nonerotic Physical Contact with Patients." *American Psychologist, 32,* pp. 843-849.

Horowitz, M. J. 1984. "Stress and the Mechanisms of Defense." In *Review of General Psychiatry,* edited by H. H. Goldman, pp. 42-50. Los Altos, Calif.: Lange Medical Publications.

_____. 1978a. *Image Formation and Cognition.* New York: Appleton-Century-Crofts.

_____. 1978b. "Controls of Visual Imagery and Therapist Intervention." In *The Power of Human Imagination: New Methods in Psychotherapy,* edited by J. L. Singer and K. S. Pope, pp. 37-49, New York: Plenum.

_____. 1976. *Stress Reponse Syndromes.* New York: Jason Aronson.

Ishida, Y. 1974. "Physician-patient Sexual Relations." *Medical Aspects of Human Sexuality, 8,* p. 103.

Jones, E. 1957. *The Life and Works of Sigmund Freud.* New York: Basic Books.

Kaplan, A. 1975. "Sex in Psychotherapy: The Myth of Sandor Ferenczi." *Contemporary Psychoanalysis, 11,* pp. 175-187.

Kaplan, D. 1972. "On Transference Love and Generativity." *Psychoanalytic Review, 58,* pp. 573-579.

Kaplan, H. S. 1977. "Training Sex Therapists." In *Ethical Issues in Sex Therapy and Research,* edited by W. H. Masters, V. E. Johnson, and R. D. Kolodny, pp. 182-205. Boston: Little, Brown.

Kardener, S. H. 1974. "Sex and the Physician-patient Relationship." *American Journal of Psychiatry, 131,* pp. 1134-1136.

Kardener, S. H., Fuller, M., and Mensh, I. N. 1976. "Characteristics of 'Erotic' Practitioners." *American Journal of Psychiatry, 133,* pp. 1324-1325.

_____. 1973. "A Survey of Physicians' Attitudes and Practices Regarding Erotic and Nonerotic Contact with Patients." *American Journal of Psychiatry, 130,* pp. 1077-1081.

Keith-Spiegel, P. C. 1979. "Sex with Clients: Ten Reasons Why It Is a Very Stupid Thing to Do." Paper presented at the annual meeting of the American Psychological Association, New York, September.

Keith-Spiegel, P. C., and Koocher, G. 1985. *Ethics in Psychology: Standards and Cases.* New York: Random House.

Kenworthy, T. A., Koufacos, C., and Sherman, J. 1976. "Women and Therapy: A Survey on Internship Programs." *Psychology of Women Quarterly, 1,* pp. 125-137.

Kernberg, O. 1975. *Borderline Conditions and Pathological Narcissism.* New York: Jason Aronson.

Kurlycheck, R., and De Heer, N. D. 1982. "Court Testimony by Mental Health Professionals in Corrections: Considerations and Guidelines for Effective Involvement." *Journal of Behavioral Technology: Methods and Training, 28,* pp. 137–139.

Laliotis, D., and Grayson, J. 1985. "Psychologist Heal Thyself: What Is Available for the Impaired Psychologist?" *American Psychologist, 40,* pp. 84–96.

Landis, C. E., Miller, H. R., and Wettstone, R. P. 1975. "Sexual Awareness Training for Counselors." *Teaching of Psychology, 2,* pp. 33–36.

Langs, R. J. 1982. "Countertransference and the Process of Cure." In *Curative Factors in Dynamic Psychotherapy,* edited by S. Slipp, pp. 127–152. New York: McGraw-Hill.

_____ . 1973. *The Technique of Psychoanalytic Psychotherapy,* Vol. 1. New York: Jason Aronson.

Lehrman, N. S. 1960. "The Analyst's Sexual Feelings." *American Journal of Psychotherapy, 14,* pp. 545–549.

Len, M., and Fischer, J. 1978. "Clinicians' Attitudes toward and Use of Four Body Contact or Sexual Techniques with Clients." *Journal of Sex Research, 14,* pp. 40–49.

Levenson, H., and Pope, K. S. 1984. "Behavior Therapy and Cognitive Therapy." In *Review of General Psychiatry,* edited by H. H. Gold, pp. 538–548. Los Altos, Calif.: Lange Medical Publications.

Lief, H. I. 1978. "Sexual Survey #7: Current Thinking on Seductive Patients." *Medical Aspects of Human Sexuality,* February, pp. 46–47.

Little, M. 1951. "Countertransference and the Patient's Response to It." *International Journal of Psychoanalysis, 32,* pp. 32–40.

Loftus, E., and Monahan, J. 1980. "Trial by Data: Psychological Research as Legal Evidence." *American Psychologist, 35,* pp. 270–283.

McCartney, J. 1966. "Overt Transference." *Journal of Sex Research, 2,* pp. 227–237.

McCormick, C. G. 1973. "If You Touch, Don't Take." *Psychotherapy: Theory, Research and Practice, 10,* pp. 199–200.

Maguire, L. 1977. "A Sex Therapist's View of Sexual Contacts." Paper presented at the annual meeting of the American Psychological Association, San Francisco, August.

Marmor, J. 1977. "Designated Discussion of 'The Ethics of Sex Therapy.'" In *Ethical Issues in Sex Therapy and Research,* edited by W. H. Masters, V. E. Johnson, and R. D. Kolodny, pp. 157–161. Boston: Little, Brown.

_____ . 1976. "Some Psychodynamic Aspects of the Seduction of Patients in Psychotherapy." *American Journal of Psychoanalysis, 36,* pp. 319–323.

_____ . 1972a. "The Seductive Psychotherapist." *Psychiatry Digest, 31,* pp. 10–16.

_____ . 1972b. "Sexual Acting Out in Psychotherapy." *The American Journal of Psychoanalysis, 32,* pp. 327–335.

_____ . 1953. "The Feeling of Superiority: An Occupational Hazard in the Practice of Psychotherapy." *American Journal of Psychiatry, 110,* pp. 3370–3373.

Masters, W. H., and Johnson, V. E. 1976. "Principles of the New Sex Therapy." *American Journal of Psychiatry, 133,* pp. 548–554.

Masterson, J. 1976. *Psychotherapy of the Borderline Adult: A Developmental Approach*. New York: Bruner/Mazel.

Mazza v. *Huffaker* 61 N.C. App. 170, 1983.

Medlicott, R. W. 1968. "Erotic Professional Indiscretions, Actual or Assumed and Alleged." *Australian/New Zealand Journal of Psychiatry, 2,* pp. 17–23.

Meichenbaum, D. 1978. "Why Does Using Imagery in Psychotherapy Lead to Change?" In *The Power of Human Imagination: New Methods of Psychotherapy,* edited by J. L. Singer and K. S. Pope, pp. 381–394. New York: Plenum.

Menninger, K. 1958. *Theory of Psychoanalytic Technique*. New York: Basic Books.

Mintz, E. E. 1969. "Touch and the Psychoanalytic Tradition." *Psychoanalytic Review, 56,* pp. 365–366.

Moldawsky, S. 1977. "Some Theoretical and Clinical Issues in Therapist-Patient Contact, or Everybody Gets Screwed and Nobody Gets Helped." Paper presented at the annual meeting of the American Psychological Association, San Francisco, August.

Morgan, H. 1977. "The Difficult Defendant: A Case Report." *American Journal of Psychiatry, 134,* pp. 1306–1307.

Morra v. *State Board of Examiners of Psychologists,* 510 P.2d 614 S.Ct. Kan. 1973.

National Association of Social Workers, Inc. 1980. "Code of Ethics of the National Association of Social Workers." Washington, D.C.

O'Byrne, B. de R. 1970. "Civil Liability of Doctor or Psychologist for Having Sexual Relationship with Patient." *American Law Reports, 33,* pp. 1393–96 and Supplement, 135.

Pakdaman, Hooshand. 1982. "The Prevalence of Sexual Intimacy between Therapists and their Clients." Unpublished doctoral dissertation, United States International University.

People v. *Bernstein,* 340 P. 2d 299, 1959.

Perry, J. A. 1976. "Physicians' Erotic and Nonerotic Involvement with Patients." *American Journal of Psychiatry, 33,* 838–840.

Plasil, E. 1985. *Therapist*. New York: St. Martin's/Marek.

Pope, K. S. In press. "Clinical and Legal Issues in Assessing and Treating the Potentially Violent Patient." *The Independent Practitioner*.

_____ . 1986a. "Assessment and Management of Suicidal Risk: Clinical and Legal Standards of Care." *The Independent Practitioner, 6*(1), pp. 17–23.

_____ . 1986b. "Therapist-Patient Sex Syndrome: Research Findings." Paper presented at the annual convention of the American Psychiatric Association, Washington, D.C., May.

_____ . 1985a. "Diagnosis and Treatment of Therapist-patient Sex Syndrome." Paper presented at the annual convention of the American Psychological Association, Los Angeles, August.

_____ . 1985b. "Fantasy." In *From Research to Clinical Practice: The Implications of Social and Developmental Research for Psychotherapy,* edited by G. Stricker and R. H. Keisner, pp. 375–400. New York: Plenum.

_____ . 1982. *Implications of Fantasy and Imagination for Mental Health: Theory, Research, and Interventions*. Report commissioned by the National Institute of Mental Health, contract number 449904865, order number 82M024784505D.

Pope, K. S., Keith-Spiegel, P. C., and Tabachnick, B. G. 1986. "Sexual Attraction to Clients: The Human Therapist and the (Sometimes) Inhuman Training System." *American Psychologist, 41,* pp. 147–158.

Pope, K. S., Levenson, H., and Schover, L. 1979. "Sexual Intimacy in Psychology Training: Results and Implications of a National Survey." *American Psychologist, 34,* pp. 682–689.

Pope, K. S., Schover, L. R., and Levenson, H. 1980. "Sexual Behavior between Clinical Supervisors and Trainees: Implications for Professional Standards." *Professional Psychology, 11,* pp. 157–162.

Rappaport, E. A. 1959. "The First Dream in an Eroticized Transference." *International Journal of Psychoanalysis, 40,* pp. 240–245.

_____ . 1956. "The Management of an Eroticized Transference." *Psychoanalytic Quarterly, 25,* pp. 515–529.

Redlich, F. C. 1977. "The Ethics of Sex Therapy." In *Ethical Issues in Sex Therapy and Research,* edited by W. H. Masters, V. E. Johnson, and R. D. Kolodny, pp. 143–157. Boston: Little, Brown.

Reich, A. 1951. "On Countertransference." *International Journal of Psychoanalysis, 32,* pp. 25–31.

Riskin, L. 1979. "Sexual Relations between Psychotherapists and their Patients: Toward Research or Restraint?" *California Law Review, 67,* pp. 1000–1027.

Robertiello, R. 1975. "Iatrogenic Psychiatric Illness." *Journal of Contemporary Psychotherapy, 7,* pp. 3–8.

Romeo, S. 1978. "Dr. Martin Shepard Answers His Accusers." *Knave,* June, pp. 14–38.

Rosenstein v. *Barnes, Superior Court of California,* L.A. County, Vase # NWC 78755, March 24, 1984.

Roy v. *Hartogs,* 381 N.Y.S. 2d 587 (App. 1976).

Ruesch, J. 1961. *Therapeutic Communication.* New York: W. W. Norton.

Sadoff, R. L. 1975. *Forensic Psychiatry: A Practical Guide for Lawyers and Psychiatrists.* Springfield, Ill.: Charles C. Thomas.

Sarason, S. B. 1985. *Caring and Compassion in Clinical Practice.* San Francisco: Jossey-Bass.

Saretsky, L. 1977. "Sex-related Countertransference Issues of a Female Therapist." *Clinical Psychologist, 30,* pp. 11–12.

Saul, L. J. 1962. "The Erotic Transference." *Psychoanalytic Quarterly, 31,* pp. 54–61.

Scheflen, A. E. 1965. "Quasi-courtship Behavior in Psychotherapy." *Psychiatry, 28,* pp. 245–257.

Schoener, G., Milgrom, J., and Gonsiorek, J. 1983. "Responding Therapeutically to Clients Who Have Been Sexually Involved With their Psychotherapists." Minneapolis: Minneapolis Walk-In Counseling Center, Monograph.

Schover, L. R. 1983. "Psychotherapists' Reactions to Client Sexuality: A source of Bias in Treatment?" In *Bias in Psychotherapy,* edited by J. Murray and P. R. Abramson, pp. 285–308. New York: Praeger.

_____ . 1981. "Male and Female Therapists' Responses to Male and Female Client Sexual Material: An Analogue Study." *Archives of Sexual Behavior, 10,* pp. 477–492.

Schultz, L. G. 1975. "Survey of Social Workers' Attitudes and Use of Body and Sexual Psychotherapies." *Clinical Social Work Journal, 3,* pp. 90–99.

Schultz, L. G., and McGrath, J. 1978. "Developing Seduction Management Skills through the Use of Video Vignettes." *Journal of Humanities, 5,* pp. 70–78.

Schutz, B. M. 1982. *Legal Liability in Psychotherapy.* San Francisco: Jossey-Bass.

Scrignar, C. 1984. *Post-Traumatic Stress Disorder.* New York: Praeger.

Seagull, A. A. 1972. "Should a Therapist Have Intercourse with Patients?" Paper presented at the annual meeting of the American Psychological Association, Honolulu, August.

Searles, H. F. 1965. "Oedipal Love in the Countertransference." In *Collected Papers on Schizophrenia and Related Subjects.* pp. 284–303. New York: International Universities Press. Original work published 1959.

Serban, G. 1981. "Sexual Activity in Therapy: Legal and Ethical Issues." *American Journal of Psychotherapy, 35,* pp. 76–85.

Shah, S. 1980. "Dangerousness: Conceptual, Prediction, and Public Policy Issues." In *Violence and the Violent Individual,* edited by R. Hays and K. Solway, pp. 151–178. New York: S.P. Medical and Scientific Books.

Shapiro, D. 1984. *Psychological Evaluation and Expert Testimony.* New York: Van Nostrand Reinhold.

Shearer, L. 1981. "Sex Between Patient and Physician." *Parade,* August 23, p. 8.

Shepard, M. 1971. *The Love Treatment: Sexual Intimacy between Patients and Psychotherapists.* New York: Wyden.

Shor, J., and Sanville, J. 1974. "Erotic Provocations and Dalliances in Psychotherapeutic Practice." *Clinical Social Work Journal, 2,* pp. 83–95.

Siassi, I., and Thomas, M. 1973. "Physicians and the New Sexual Freedom." *American Journal of Psychiatry, 130,* pp. 1256–1257.

Siegel, S. 1983. Personal Communication.

Simon, R. 1985. "Sexual Misconduct of Therapists: A Cause for Civil and Criminal Action." *Trial,* May, pp. 46–51.

Singer, E. 1970. *Key Concepts in Psychotherapy.* New York: Basic Books.

Singer, J. L. 1974. *Imagery and Daydream Methods in Psychotherapy and Behavior Modification.* New York: Academic Press.

Singer, J. L., and Pope, K. S. 1978. "The Use of Imagery and Fantasy Techniques in Psychotherapy." In *The Power of Human Imagination: New Methods in Psychotherapy,* edited by J. L. Singer and K. S. Pope, pp. 3–34. New York: Plenum.

Sinnett, R., and Linford, O. 1982. "Processing Formal Complaints against Psychologists." *Psychological Reports, 50,* pp. 535–544.

Smith, R. 1980. "Overview of State Medical Society Programs." *Proceedings of the Fourth AMA Conference on the Impaired Physician: Building Well-Being,* edited by J. J. Robertson, pp. 3–7, Chicago: American Medical Association.

Smith, S. 1981. "Analytic Explorations of Therapists involved with Patients." Paper presented to the annual meeting of the California State Psychological Association, San Diego, February.

Solloway v. *Department of Professional Regulation,* 421 So. 2d 573, 1982.

Sonne, J. L. (in press.) "Therapist/Patient Sexual Intimacy: Understanding and Counseling the Patient." *Medical Aspects of Human Sexuality.*

Sonne, J., Meyer, C. B., Borys, D., and Marshall, V. 1985. "Clients' Reactions to Sexual Intimacy in Therapy." *American Journal of Orthopsychiatry, 55,* pp. 183–189.

Spitz, R. 1956. "Transference: The Analytic Setting and its Prototype." *International Journal of Psychoanalysis, 37,* pp. 380–385.

Stekel, W. 1926. *Frigidity in Women in Relation to Her Love Life.* New York: Boni and Liveright.

Stone, A. A. 1983. "Sexual Misconduct by Psychiatrists: The Ethical and Clinical Dilemma of Confidentiality." *American Journal of Psychiatry, 140,* pp. 195–197.

_____ . 1976. "The Legal Implications of Sexual Activity between Psychiatrist and Patient." *American Journal of Psychiatry, 113,* pp. 1138–1141.

Stone, L. G. 1980. "A Study of the Relationships among Anxious Attachment, Ego Functioning, and Female Patients' Vulnerability to Sexual Involvement with their Male Psychotherapists." Unpublished doctoral dissertation, California School of Professional Psychology, Los Angeles.

Stone, M. H. 1982. "Turning Points in Psychotherapy." In *Curative Factors in Dynamic Psychotherapy,* edited by S. Slipp, pp. 259–279. New York: McGraw-Hill.

_____ . 1976. "Boundary Violations between Therapist and Patient." *Psychiatric Annals, 6,* pp. 8–31.

Tauber, E. S. 1979. "Countertransference Reexamined." In *Countertransference,* edited by L. Epstein and A. H. Feiner, pp. 59–70. New York: Jason Aronson.

Taylor, B. J., and Wagner, N. W. 1976. "Sex between Therapists and Clients: A Review and Analysis." *Professional Psychology, 7,* pp. 593–601.

Thompson, C. 1950. *Psychoanalysis: Evolution and Development,* New York: Hermitage House.

_____ . 1946. "Transference as a Therapeutic Instrument." In *Current Therapies of Personality Disorders,* edited by B. Gluck, pp. 194–205. New York: Grune and Stratton.

Tower, L. E. 1956. "Countertransference." *Journal of the American Psychoanalytic Association, 4,* pp. 224–255.

Turkington, C. 1984, December. "Women Therapists Not Immune to Sexual Involvement Suits." *APA Monitor, 15,* p. 15.

Ulanov, A. B. 1979. "Follow-up Treatment in Cases of Patient-Therapist Sex." *Journal of the American Academy of Psychoanalysis, 7,* pp. 101-110.

Van Buren, A. 1978. "Dear Abby." San Francisco *Sunday Examiner and Chronicle,* June 11, p. 6.

VandenBos, G. R., and Stapp, J. 1983. "Service Providers in Psychology: Results of the 1982 APA Human Resources Survey." *American Psychologist, 38,* pp. 1330–1352.

Vinson, J. S. 1984. "Sexual Contact with Psychotherapists: A Study of Client Reactions and Complaint Procedures." Unpublished doctoral dissertation, California School of Professional Psychology.

Voth, H. M. "Love Affair Between Doctor and Patient." *American Journal of Psychotherapy, 26,* pp. 394–400.

Walker, E., and Young, T. D. 1986. *A Killing Cure.* New York: Henry Holt.

Weiner, M. F. 1978. *Therapist Disclosure: The Use of Self in Psychotherapy.* Woburn, Mass.: Butterworths.

Weisstub, D. 1977. "Confidentiality and the Mental Health Professional." *Canadian Psychiatric Association Journal, 22,* pp. 319–323.

Whitesell v. *Green,* Hawaii District Court, Honolulu Docket No. 38745, November 19, 1973.

Winnicott, D. 1949. "Hate in the Countertransference." *International Journal of Psychoanalysis, 30,* pp. 69–75.

Wolowitz, H. 1972. "Hysterical Character and Feminine Identity." In *Readings on the Psychology of Women,* edited by R. Bardwick, pp. 307–314. New York: Harper and Row.

_____ . 1970. "Hysterical Character and Feminine Identity." In *Readings on the Psychology of Women,* edited by R. Bardwick, pp. 307–314. New York: Harper and Row.

Wright, R. W. 1981. "Psychologists and Professional Liability Malpractice Insurance: A Retrospective Review." *American Psychologist, 36,* pp. 1485–1493.

Zieke, Paul. 1985. "Judge Urged to Resign After Child Rape Decision." Los Angeles *Herald Examiner,* July 18, p. A6.

Zipkin v. *Freeman,* 436 S.W. 2d 753 Mo. 1968.

Ziskin, J. 1984a. *Coping with Psychiatric and Psychological Testimony,* third edition. Volumes I and II. Venice, Calif.: Law and Psychology Press.

_____ . 1984b. "Malingering of Psychological Disorders." *Behavioral Sciences and the Law, 2,* 39–49.

Index

abusive relationships, 50
acting out, 18
acting-out behavior, 39
adjudication, 143
administrative hearings, 127, 143
administrative law process, 161–63
adversarial process, 138
advocacy groups, 70–74
advocacy for patients, by subsequent
     therapists, 70
agencies, 152–54
alcohol abuse, 41
Alcoholics Anonymous, 40
alienation, 62
alienation of affections, 130
Alzheimers syndrome, 23
ambivalence, 92–95
American Association for Marriage
     and Family Therapy, 115
American Association of State
     Psychology Boards, 159, 162
American Association of Suicidology,
     18
American Medical Association (AMA),
     40, 115, 156
American Psychiatric Association, 23,
     54, 150
American Psychoanalytic Association,
     115
American Psychological Association,
     1, 115, 150; Ethics Committee,
     38, 75, 154
anger, 95–97; repressed, 95; suppres-
     sed, 95
anti-heart-balm statutes, 130
antipsychotic drugs, 55
anxiety attacks, 50
Association of American Trial Law-
     yers, 133
attention, impairment of, 105
attorney-client relationship, 124
attorney retainment, complaint filing
     and, 119

autonomous ego functioning, 52
autonomy, of patient, 89–90

babiturates, 55
battered spouses, 2
Bazelon, Judge, 139
Bernstein v. *Board of Medical Examin-
     ers, 127*
Betrayal, 25, 92, 112, 118, 146, 154,
     155
biases, 84, 113
Birkner v. *Michael Flowers and Salt
     Lake County, 152*
Birth of a Nation, 113
body-mind integration, 13
"Burning Bed, The," 154
burnout, 44

California State Psychological Associa-
     tion, 156
case value, 133–34
child abuse, 2, 53; mandatory report-
     ing laws and, 83
child neglect, due to trauma, 66
civil action(s), 128; defense to, 131–33
civil courts, 143
civil litigation, 127
civil rights, abridgement of, 92
clarity of roles, 89–90
client goals, 126
cocaine, 13
cognitive-behavioral technique, 106
cognitive dysfunction, 105
cognitive functioning, disruption of,
     62
colleague consultation, 1
*Colorado State Board of Medical Ex-
     aminers* v. *Weiler, 127*
communication, 89–90
complaint process: attorneys and,
     121–35; mental health profes-
     sionals and, 136–49; patient and,
     110–20

About the Authors

KENNETH S. POPE is a Clinical Diplomate (American Board of Professional Psychology) and a licensed psychologist in independent practice. He received his M.A. in English Literature from Harvard University, where he was a Woodrow Wilson Fellow, and his Ph.D. in clinical psychology from Yale University. Former Chair of the Ethics Committee of the California State Psychological Association, he is currently a member of the Ethics Committee of the American Psychological Association. A recipient of the Silver Psi Award of the California State Psychological Association and also of the Belle Meyer Bromberg Award for Literature, he is coeditor of the journal *Imagination, Cognition, and Personality*. Cofounder of the UCLA Post-Therapy Support Group, he has specialized in clinical work and research regarding therapist-patient and student-teacher sexual intimacy. His previous books include *The Stream of Consciousness: Scientific Investigations into the Flow of Human Experience, The Power of Human Imagination: New Methods of Psychotherapy* (both coedited with Jerome L. Singer), and *On Love and Loving: Psychological Perspectives on the Nature and Experience of Romantic Love.*

JACQUELINE C. BOUHOUTSOS is a clinical psychologist in independent practice and a Clinical Professor of Psychology at UCLA. She received a Master's degree in Social Work from the University of California at Berkeley and her Ph.D. in clinical psychology from the University of Innsbruck, Austria. For the last eight years she has specialized in working with patients who have been sexually involved with their therapists and has authored a number of research studies on this topic. Cofounder of the Post-Therapy Support Group at the UCLA Psychology Clinic, Dr. Bouhoutsos has served on ethics, standards, and peer review committees and is currently Ethics Chair of the California State Psychological Association. Former president of that association, she is also a member of the Council of Representatives of the American Psychological Association. Her professional interests include media psychology and other areas of community psychology.